T0205383

Pathological Voice Analysis

David Zhang • Kebin Wu

Pathological Voice Analysis

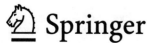 Springer

David Zhang (iD)
The Chinese University
of Hong Kong (Shenzhen)
Shenzhen Institute of Artificial
Intelligence and Robotics for Society
Guangdong, China

Kebin Wu
Huawei Technologies
Beijing, China

ISBN 978-981-32-9198-0   ISBN 978-981-32-9196-6   (eBook)
https://doi.org/10.1007/978-981-32-9196-6

© Springer Nature Singapore Pte Ltd. 2020
This work is subject to copyright. All rights are reserved by the Publisher, whether the whole or part of the material is concerned, specifically the rights of translation, reprinting, reuse of illustrations, recitation, broadcasting, reproduction on microfilms or in any other physical way, and transmission or information storage and retrieval, electronic adaptation, computer software, or by similar or dissimilar methodology now known or hereafter developed.
The use of general descriptive names, registered names, trademarks, service marks, etc. in this publication does not imply, even in the absence of a specific statement, that such names are exempt from the relevant protective laws and regulations and therefore free for general use.
The publisher, the authors, and the editors are safe to assume that the advice and information in this book are believed to be true and accurate at the date of publication. Neither the publisher nor the authors or the editors give a warranty, expressed or implied, with respect to the material contained herein or for any errors or omissions that may have been made. The publisher remains neutral with regard to jurisdictional claims in published maps and institutional affiliations.

This Springer imprint is published by the registered company Springer Nature Singapore Pte Ltd.
The registered company address is: 152 Beach Road, #21-01/04 Gateway East, Singapore 189721, Singapore

Preface

The human voice contains rich information about the speaker, such as identity, gender, health, situation, and emotion. However, the biomedical value of voice is less addressed compared with its biometrics applications such as speech recognition and speaker identification. In this book, we present the importance and value of voice in aiding diagnosis through pathological voice analysis.

We systematically introduce our research works on pathological voice analysis from the following three aspects: (1) a review on pathological voice analysis and a guideline on voice acquisition for clinical application; (2) design appropriate signal processing algorithms for pathological voice; and (3) extract biomedical information in voice to improve disease detection, such as dictionary-based feature learning and multi-audio fusion. Experimental results have shown the superiority of these techniques. These proposed methods can be used in applications of voice quality assessment, disease detection, disease severity prediction, and even the analysis of other similar signals. This book will be useful to researchers, professionals, and postgraduate students working in the field of speech signal processing, pattern recognition, biomedical engineering, etc. This book also will be very meaningful for interdisciplinary research.

The book is organized as follows: In Chap. 1, the development of pathological voice analysis is systematically reviewed. Then important factors in the acquisition of pathological voice, sampling rate in particular, are discussed in Chap. 2. After that, two of the widely used signal processing steps in pathological voice analysis, which are pitch estimation and glottal closure instant (GCI) detection, are studied in Chaps. 3 and 4, respectively. In Chap. 5, feature learning based on spherical K-means is proposed, in contrast to the traditional handcrafted features. In Chaps. 6 and 7, we investigate multi-audio fusion in pathological voice analysis so as to make full use of the multiple audios collected for each subject. Finally, we summarize the book and give a short introduction to future works that may contribute to the further development of pathological voice analysis in Chap. 8.

Our team has been working on pathological voice analysis for more than 5 years. We appreciate the related grant supports from the GRF fund of the HKSAR

Government, Research projects from Shenzhen Institutes of both Big Data and Artificial Intelligence & Robotics for Society, and the National Natural Science Foundation of China (NSFC) (61020106004, 61332011, 61272292, and 61271344). Besides, we thank Prof. Guangming Lu and Prof. Zhenhua Guo for their valuable suggestions about our research on pathological voice analysis.

Guangdong, China   David Zhang
Beijing, China   Kebin Wu
April 2020

Contents

Chapter 1
Introduction

Abstract Recently, computer-based pathological voice analysis has become increasingly popular. This chapter first discusses the necessity for the study of pathological voice analysis, and then a systematic review is presented, including the diseases which may lead to pathological voice, current development of pathological voice analysis in the aspects of voice recording, feature extraction, and classification (regression). Finally, the key problems and challenges in pathological voice analysis are discussed. After reading this chapter, people will have some shallow ideas on pathological voice analysis.

Keywords Pathological voice analysis · Disease detection · Disease monitoring

Recently, computer-based pathological voice analysis has become increasingly popular. This chapter first discusses the necessity for the study of pathological voice analysis, and then a systematic review is presented, including the diseases which may lead to pathological voice, current development of pathological voice analysis in the aspects of voice recording, feature extraction, and classification (regression). Finally, the key problems and challenges in pathological voice analysis are discussed. After reading this chapter, people will have some shallow ideas on pathological voice analysis.

1.1 Pathological Voice Analysis

In this book, voice refers to all possible sounds produced by the human vocal system, such as vowels, continuous speech, and coughing sounds. While studying voice has always been a great interest for researchers from various fields, we mainly focus on the voice analysis in the fields of machine learning and signal processing in this book.

In recent years, speaker and speech recognition are two main applications that adopt machine learning technique on voice. In speaker recognition, voice pronounced by a speaker is termed as a biometric signal including identity related characteristic so that it can be used to recognize the identity of the speaker (Kinnunen and Li 2010). Speech recognition, however, is to recognize and translate spoken language into text (Rabiner 1989). In both cases, signal processing (such as de-noising (Milone et al. 2010) and pitch estimation (Atal 1972)) and machine learning technique (Miro et al. 2012; Graves et al. 2013) play significant roles.

Unlike speaker and speech recognition which has been widely studied and even adopted in industry extensively, the biomedical value of voice is less emphasized. The production of voice requires the cooperation of multiple organs: (1) the nervous system that coordinates the operation of various tissues and organs in the process of voice production; (2) the respiratory system that provides energy, including lungs and tracheas; and (3) the vocal cords and vocal tracts that function as vibrators and resonators, respectively. When a certain disease affects either of the three abovementioned system directly or indirectly, pathological voice may be generated. For example, studies have shown that voice quantitative analysis can be used to detect neurological diseases such as Alzheimer's disease (AD) (López-de-Ipiña et al. 2013), Parkinson's disease (PD) (Tsanas 2012), and stroke (Le et al. 2014). When suffered from respiratory diseases such as lung cancer and chronic obstructive pneumonia, patients may catch on symptoms like dysphonia and cough (Lee et al. 2008). In addition, organic lesions occurring in vocal cord and tract can lead to hoarse voice. For example, Saudi et al. classified healthy voice and voice collected from patients with vocal cord nodules, abscesses, polyps, paralysis, edema, and vocal cord cancer with an accuracy of 92.86% (Saudi et al. 2012). Therefore, pathological voice analysis can be used to help diagnose (even monitor) the healthy status of vocal system.

In clinical applications, however, there exist many alternative methods to diagnose diseases that affect voice. Hence, the necessity of pathological voice analysis is furthermore clarified. Firstly, comparing with common medical signals such as electroencephalogram (EEG) and electrocardiogram (ECG), voice signal collection does not need special acquisition devices. For instance, Little et al. of Oxford University launched a PVI (Parkinson's voice initiative) to collect voices of 10,000 Parkinson's patients worldwide in order to realize Parkinson's disease detection and monitoring based on voice analysis. In this initiative, the signal acquisition device is by telephone which is quite ubiquitous. Secondly, pathological voice analysis is user-friendly, painless, and non-invasive. Traditional laryngoscopy in diagnosis inserts a tubular endoscope into the larynx through the mouth to observe the interior of the larynx, which may cause nausea and vomiting in patients and lead to lesion due to the friction between instruments and skin, mucosa, tissues, and organs. Besides, unqualified sterilization and anesthesia are also high-risk factors. In contrast, collecting voice is a non-invasive and painless process so that patients may be more actively involved in voice acquisition. Thirdly, voice analysis may be the key method for the early detection of some certain diseases. Rusza et al. found that most patients with early Parkinson's disease had some degree of speech disorder and it often appeared earlier than other symptoms like dyskinesia (Rusz et al. 2011). At present, the cause of Parkinson's disease (PD) is not completely understood by researchers and there is no radical cure for the disease. If patients can get treatment at the early stage of PD onset, the development of the disease can be delayed (King et al. 1994). Therefore, if people with high-risk of PD can be screened regularly based on voice analysis, it is possible to detect the disease as soon as possible so as to obtain early treatment. Fourthly, disease diagnosis and monitoring by voice analysis is automatic and objective. In recent years, the traditional diagnosis and monitoring of Parkinson's disease is mainly decided by a doctor subjectively based on the patient's medical history, self-description of symptoms, and the reaction to certain drugs (such as levodopa). Besides, brain computed tomography (CT), magnetic resonance imaging (MRI), and positron emission tomography (PET) are also employed to exclude some similar diseases. Obviously, the widely used diagnostic method relies too much on doctors, and thus the diagnostic results are possible to be affected by doctors' medical skills, emotions, and physical state. In contrast, objective voice analysis can improve the reliability of initial diagnosis and follow-up: in diagnosis, objective measurement and analysis of patient's voice offer more accurate information so as to reduce the rate of missed diagnosis and misdiagnosis; in follow-up, objective voice analysis method provides the basis for doctors to adjust the patients' dosage reasonably. For example, Tsanas et al. established a Parkinson's disease detection model based on voice analysis and obtained an accuracy of 98.5 ($\pm 2.3\%$) (Tsanas 2012). At the same time, the author extended the application of voice analysis to the severity prediction of PD (Tsanas 2012). In addition, Wang Jianqun's research showed that the objective analysis of pathological voice can also be used to effectively evaluate the effect of surgery (Wang et al. 2004). Fifth, voice analysis can promote the development of telemedicine. Traditional diagnostic methods require face-to-face contact between patients and doctors and patients need to visit hospitals frequently for follow-up, which will bring great inconvenience to the elderly, especially those with disabilities such as PD and stroke. On the contrary, the objective voice measurement does not require the direct participation of doctors so that patients are expected to get diagnosis and severity prediction at home, eliminating the inconvenience of visiting hospitals. Moreover, the convenience of objective voice analysis enables patients to make quantitative measurements at home many times a day. The timely and frequent measurements enable doctors to give more appropriate and reasonable treatment plans accordingly. Sixth, voice analysis is highly cost-effective. The low cost of voice acquisition and analysis makes it possible for more patients to obtain early detection, early treatment, and regular follow-up. Finally, voice analysis may improve the life quality for patients. It is well known that patients with pathological voice often present certain obstacles in communication, which affect their quality of life. Song et al. analyzed the spectral characteristics of pathological voice and proposed a voice enhancement algorithm to reduce the wheezing in patients' voice without losing biometric characteristics (Song et al. 2013).

1.2   Computerized Voice Analysis

The biomedical significance of voice is less emphasized compared with its other applications, such as speaker recognition and speech recognition. This section presents a review of the computerized voice analysis in biomedical field so that the biomedical value of voice can be reemphasized. Firstly, we show by a literature review that many diseases result in pathological voice and these diseases are categorized into three classes based on the voice production mechanism: nerve system diseases, respiratory system diseases, and diseases in vocal folds and vocal tract. Secondly, the three steps in computerized voice analysis, which are voice recording, feature extraction, and classification and regression, are reviewed separately to show the current development of voice analysis in the biomedical field. Finally, the potential challenges to be addressed in computerized voice analysis are discussed in terms of data level and algorithm level. Some suggestions concerning future research direction are also presented. Computerized voice analysis is a promising complementary tool for disease diagnosis and monitoring; however, there are several inevitable challenges to be handled before it is put into practical use.

1.2.1   Introduction

Health related studies are bringing along a growth of attention from governmental agencies, charities, and companies since diseases pose increasing social and economic burdens on society (The US Burden of Disease Collaborators 2018; Milken Institute 2018). Technologies from different fields are often adopted to assist the research. One of them is to utilize the modern computerized technique since it possesses two advantages: (1) automation that helps to reduce manual labor and (2) objectiveness which enables the detection and monitoring of disease less dependent on the doctors' expertise. This section presents a literature review of biomedical analysis of voice that is based on computerized technology. Even though voice is one kind of biomedical signal, its biomedical value is far less emphasized than its other applications, such as speaker recognition and speech recognition. Hence, this review aims to reemphasize the significance of voice in the biomedical field and discuss the accompanied challenges.

As shown in Titze (1994) and (Mekyska et al. 2015), the term voice can be defined in both a broad and a narrow sense. While it refers to the sound in which the vocal folds vibrate in the narrow sense, voice may be taken as synonymous of speech in the broad sense. In this section, we take the broad definition and sounds pronounced by a human being, such as simple vowels, continuous speech, and cough, are all included. Voice, as a biomedical signal, is generated under the cooperation of multiple systems and diseases in these systems often show abnormality in voice. The commercial database MEEI (Massachusetts Eye and Ear Infirmary) (Elemetrics 1994) developed by Massachusetts Eye and Ear Infirmary Voice & Speech Lab is frequently exploited to analyze pathological voices. In this dataset, voices of laryngeal diseases are included, such as vocal fold polyp, adductor spasmodic dysphonia, keratosis leukoplakia, vocal nodules, and vocal fold paralysis. In recent decades, studies suggest that voice analysis can also be used to detect and monitor some neurological disorders, such as Alzheimer's disease (AD) (Lopez-de Ipina et al. 2013) and Parkinson's disease (PD) (Tsanas et al. 2010, 2012; Little et al. 2009; Rusz et al. 2011; Mandal and Sairam 2013; Tsanas 2012; Little 2007). Diseases related to respiratory system can also result in pathological voice. In Lee et al. (2008), it was pointed out that 90% of lung cancer patients were perceived as dysphonic. Finally, pathological voice can be generated indirectly. Renal failure, for example, affects voice by generating disturbances in the respiratory system (Kumar and Bhat 2010; Hamdan et al. 2005; Jung et al. 2014).

In spite of these studies, there are few summaries to clarify the biomedical value of voice. In this work, we aim to reemphasize the biomedical value of voice. Firstly, a review of the existing literature is provided to demonstrate that lots of diseases lead to abnormal voices. Besides, these diseases are classified into three categories according to the mechanism of voice production. Secondly, three steps in computerized voice analysis in biomedical applications are reviewed separately, offering a basic summary of its present situation. Thirdly, we discuss the potential challenges to be handled in computerized voice analysis from both data level and algorithm level. Additionally, we also present some suggestions concerning future research direction on computerized voice analysis.

The remainder of this section is organized as follows. In Sect. 1.2.2, a literature review is presented showing that many diseases affect voice and these diseases can be categorized into three classes, according to the mechanism of voice production. In Sect. 1.2.3, we review the present situations for the three steps in computerized voice analysis separately. Section 1.2.4 presents the discussion of potential challenges in the computerized voice analysis from both data and algorithm level. Suggestions concerning future research directions are also included. Conclusions are given in Sect. 1.2.5.

1.2.2 Biomedical Value of Voice

Recently, there have been more and more studies analyzing the pathological voice, as can be seen in Fig. 1.1. Various diseases can lead to pathological voice. In this section, the biomedical value of voice is reemphasized by literature review and the diseases resulting in pathological voice are categorized. The reviewed literature use voice as a biomedical signal and adopt computer-aided technology to implement analysis.

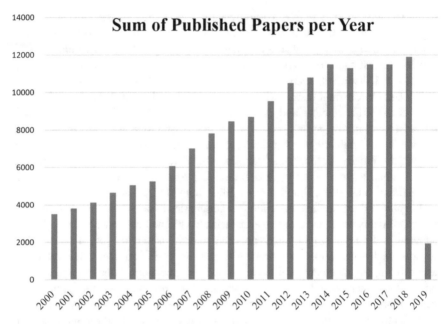

Fig. 1.1 The number of published papers on the topic of pathological voice analysis. The numbers were obtained by searching "pathological voice analysis" in Google Scholar on March 22, 2019

1.2.2.1　Mechanism of Voice Production

Before the review, we present a brief description of how voice is produced, aiming to show the organs involved in phonation.

Air flowing is an essential part of voice production. The airflow first originates from lungs, goes up along trachea to larynx, and then exits from mouth and nose. Systems involved in this process can be classified into three categories depending on their functions: (1) The nerve system coordinates the interactions of involved systems in voice production: (2) The respiratory system, including lungs and trachea, is regarded as the energy source (Tsanas 2012; David 2010); (3) vocal cords and vocal tract are called as vibrator and resonator, respectively. When producing a voiced sound, vocal cords are driven by airflow from respiratory system to open and close repeatedly, forming vibrations. Vocal tract, which is assumed as a tube formed by several anatomical segments: pharynx, oral cavity, nasal cavity, and soft palate changes its shape flexibly with different syllables to form resonance (Titze 1994).

With the coordination of the three abovementioned systems, voice can be produced. When a disease occurs in these systems, pathological voice may be generated.

1.2.2.2 Voice and Diseases

Diseases that affect voice can be grouped into three classes, according to the categorization of involved systems in voice production in Sect. 1.2.2.1.

Voice and Diseases in Nerve System

In this category, three typical diseases affect voice, which are Alzheimer's disease (AD), Parkinson's disease (PD), and stroke.

AD patients are often featured with progressive cognitive deterioration. Most of them have difficulty in communicating and their emotional responses are impaired. These characteristics show signs in voice. Therefore, it was proposed to extract quantitative features from voice for early diagnosis of AD. For instance, the Automatic Spontaneous Speech Analysis (ASSA) and Emotional Response Analysis (ERA) on speech were employed to diagnose Alzheimer's disease (AD) as well as to predict its severity degree in Lopez-de Ipina et al. (2013).

PD is another neurodegenerative disorder resulting in voice impairment and there have been varieties of literature showing that voice analysis is one effective non-invasive way for PD diagnosis (Tsanas et al. 2010, 2012; Little et al. 2009; Rusz et al. 2011; Mandal and Sairam 2013; Tsanas 2012; Little 2007) and monitoring (Tsanas et al. 2011; Wang et al. 2016; Arora et al. 2015). As pointed out in Tsanas et al. (2012), PD leads to the malfunction of nerve systems, making the cooperation of organs in voice production less appropriate and delicate. The produced voice is hoarse, breathy, less articulated and the prosody aspect of voice is shown as monoloudness, reduction of stress, and monopitch (Schulz and Grant 2000). Based on this observation, Tsanas (2012) conducted voice analysis to detect PD and the accuracy rate reported was $98.5 \pm 2.3\%$. It should be highly stressed that abnormality in the voice is often shown earlier than other symptoms (Harel et al. 2004), making voice analysis more important for the early diagnosis of PD. In addition, Tsanas also made progresses in predicting the symptom severity of PD, which is often described by the Unified Parkinson's Disease Rating Scale (UPDRS). The reported mean absolute error in predicting UPDRS by regression based on voice features was 1.59 ± 0.17 (UPDRS ranges from 0 to 176) (Tsanas 2012). In Garcia et al. (2017), the i-vector framework was utilized to model the speech of PD patients and thus to predict their neurological state. These experimental results show that it is promising to use computerized voice analysis for PD detection and monitoring. Actually, there is a project, named as Parkinson's Voice Initiative (Tsanas and Little 2012), aiming to collect large numbers of voice samples from healthy volunteers and PD patients. With this large database, the model of voice analysis can be further optimized for PD detection and monitoring. Readers may refer to the work in Benba (2016) for another review on voice based PD assessment.

Stroke disease often leads to aphasia. Patients with aphasia have difficulty in communication, i.e., speaking rate is slow and the speech length tends to be short.

Thus, speech signals have been employed for stroke monitoring. In Le et al. (2014), a system was devised to assess the speech quality of patients with aphasia objectively, using acoustical measures such as voiced duration and the rate of clear speech over all speech. Similarly, another automatic system for detecting voice disorders, particularly for stroke, was presented in Brauers et al. (2006). This system was designed for home use, making it especially useful for patients during stroke rehabilitation and those with suspicious symptoms of stroke.

A patient with any of these diseases often suffers from a shorter life span and impacted life quality. When literature evidence showing that automatic voice analysis is promising for the detection and monitoring of these diseases, voice analysis needs more attention.

Voice and Diseases in Respiratory System

A malfunctioning respiratory system shows signs in voice. For instance, cough is a common symptom and its frequency, strength, and other characteristics of cough can be used to screen respiratory diseases (Shrivastav et al. 2014). In Lee et al. (2008), it was pointed out that 90% of the lung cancer patients are perceived as dysphonic. An acoustical analysis for the chronic obstructive pulmonary disease (COPD) was carried out in Shastry et al. (2014) and the experimental results showed that the values of acoustical measures extracted from patients with COPD and healthy subjects, respectively, were significantly different.

In addition to diseases affecting respiration systems directly, illness originating from other organs can influence the produced voice indirectly. One main concern is the renal failure disease, which leads to disturbances in the pulmonary system and the voices of patients often have increased pitch (Kumar and Bhat 2010). Experiments demonstrated that the acoustical differences between patients with renal failure and healthy controls were significant and the underlying pathophysiology for the differences was explained in Kumar and Bhat (2010). In Hamdan et al. (2005) and Jung et al. (2014), the effects of hemodialysis, which is a typical treatment for renal failure, on voice were investigated. Cystic fibrosis (CF) disease is another disease affecting voice indirectly and it generates drastic respiratory symptoms such as short breathiness and chronic coughing. In Louren et al. (2014), experimental results demonstrated that acoustical features measuring deviations of vocal parameters display significant differences between CF patients and the control group.

Since dysfunction of the respiration system often causes chronic cough, shorter breath, and even death in severe case, an effective and non-invasive monitoring tool will bring convenience. The studies indicate that acoustical analysis may be one promising solution.

Voice and Diseases in Vocal Folds and Vocal Tract

Diseases in vocal folds and tract have direct impacts on voice. In fact, studies that use voice for biomedical purposes are primarily focused on diseases in this category. Besides, computerized voice analysis system has been put into practical use in the ENT (ear, nose, and throat) department of many hospitals.

Among all systems involved during voice production, vocal folds are the most sensitive tissue (Arjmandi and Pooyan 2012). It was pointed out in Akbari and Arjmandi (2014) that vocal folds, along with vocal tract, are the most important components so that voice can be highly influenced by diseases in these systems. In Campisi et al. (2000), the voice pattern for patients with vocal cord nodules was analyzed. It was demonstrated in Oguz et al. (2007) that unilateral vocal cord paralysis, another disease in vocal folds, had effects on acoustic measures. Besides, many literature treat voices of multiple diseases as a single class and attempt to distinguish them from normal voices (Dibazar et al. 2002; Godino-Llorente et al. 2006; Henrıquez et al. 2009; Markaki and Stylianou 2009, 2011; Parsa and Jamieson 2000). Study in Saudi et al. (2012) showed that healthy subjects could be discriminated from patients with six vocal fold diseases, including cyst, polyps, nodules, paralysis, edemas, and carcinoma by acoustical analysis, with an accuracy of 92.86%. In Akbari and Arjmandi (2014), three other diseases affecting the vibration function of vocal folds were analyzed. More types of vocal folds diseases resulting in pathological voices can be found in the widely used database (MEEI Elemetrics 1994). Literature concerning voice analysis for diagnosis of vocal folds diseases fall into two classes. On one hand, some aim to screen pathological voices by treating voices of several vocal folds diseases as one group and comparing extracted acoustical measurements with that of normal voices (Dibazar et al. 2002; Godino-Llorente et al. 2006; Henrıquez et al. 2009; Hadjitodorov and Mitev 2002; Vikram and Umarani 2013; Boyanov and Hadjitodorov 1997; Saeedi et al. 2011; Arjmandi et al. 2011). On the other hand, there are some research attempting to use voice to identify the type of vocal folds diseases (Markaki and Stylianou 2009; Arjmandi and Pooyan 2012; Jothilakshmi 2014; Alsulaiman 2014; Cavalcanti et al. 2010). Arjmandi and Pooyan presented an algorithm to classify six different voice disorders: paralysis, nodules, polyp, edema, spasmodic dysphonia, and keratosis (disease in the vocal tract) (Arjmandi and Pooyan 2012). Likewise, the automatic system developed in Jothilakshmi (2014) was designed to classify ten types of diseases by voice analysis.

Three main elements determining the shape of vocal tract are tongue, nose cavity, and oral cavity. Disease in these three places can lead to unnatural shape change of vocal tract and thus abnormal voice is generated. Oral, head, and neck cancer (OHNC), which includes any cancer starting in the upper digestive tract (Zhou et al. 2012), often affects vocal tract severely and consequently leads to degraded speech intelligibility. Experiments in Maier et al. (2009) proved that the speech intelligibility of OHNC patients was significantly worse than that of the control group by analyzing with an automatic speech recognition system (ASR). Besides, there are investigations implemented to compare the acoustical parameter changes

Table 1.1 The summarized list of diseases affecting voice

Classes	Typical diseases
Nerve system	AD (Lopez-de Ipina et al. 2013); PD (Tsanas 2012); Stroke (Brauers et al. 2006)
Respiratory system	Lung cancer (Lee et al. 2008); COPD (Shastry et al. 2014); Renal failure (Kumar and Bhat 2010); Cystic fibrosis (Louren et al. 2014)
Vocal folds and vocal tract	Paralysis (Saudi et al. 2012); Nodules (Saudi et al. 2012); Polyp (Saudi et al. 2012); Edema (Saudi et al. 2012); Spasmodic dysphonia (Arjmandi et al. 2011); Keratosis (Arjmandi et al. 2011); OHNC (Maier et al. 2009); Leukoplakia (Saeedi and Almasganj 2013); Acute rhinitis (Lee et al. 2005); CLP (Orozco-Arroyave et al. 2011); Nasal obstruction (Lee et al. 2005)

before and after treatments for OHNC (Whitehill et al. 2006; De Bruijn et al. 2009). Leukoplakia is another vocal tract disease with abnormal voices (Saeedi and Almasganj 2013). Additionally, some diseases, such as acute rhinitis (nasal allergy), cleft lip and palate (CLP), and nasal obstruction, show hypernasality in voice (Lee et al. 2005; Orozco-Arroyave et al. 2011) and acoustical features to detect hypernasality can be found in Orozco-Arroyave et al. (2011) and Castellanos et al. (2006).

Voice assessment is also meaningful for diseases affecting vocal folds indirectly. For instance, thyroid patients sometimes suffer from vocal dysfunction, and acoustic measurements for thyroid patients and the control group have distinct differences (Orozco-Arroyave et al. 2011). Furthermore, voice analysis is a useful tool to monitor the rehabilitation after thyroid surgery (Orozco-Arroyave et al. 2011). In sum, three categories of diseases may show signs in voice, as summarized in Table 1.1.

Necessity of Computerized Voice Analysis

Traditionally, most diseases in Table 1.1 are usually diagnosed by doctors, with the help of specially designed tools like laryngoscope, stroboscope, and endoscope (Arjmandi and Pooyan 2012). The current diagnostic methods have disadvantages such as high costs, requiring specialist, and being invasive. In addition, the morbidity rates of diseases in vocal folds and tract are relatively high, especially for teachers (Roy et al. 2004; Williams 2014). Hence, alternative approaches should be investigated to overcome the current limitations.

In Sect. 1.2.2.2, the potential of computerized voice analysis for diagnosis and monitoring of diseases that influence the articulatory-related systems is reviewed. The appealing merits of computerized voice analysis, such as low cost, high convenience, no pain, and no invasion, may help to decrease the burden of both hospitals and patients and thus may become a complementary tool to the current diagnostic and monitoring methods, even though wide clinical use is still a long way to go. Clearly, the biomedical value of voice is reemphasized in this section.

1.2.3 Present Situation of Computerized Voice Analysis

When computerized voice analysis is used for disease diagnosis and monitoring, the first step is to record voices from patients, followed by the calculations of acoustical objective measurements. Then the measurements are used as features for classification (for diagnosis) or regression (for monitoring). In this section, the current situation of each stage is presented in brief.

1.2.3.1 Voice Database

Voice database is indispensable for acoustical analysis. However, many databases in the literature of computerized voice analysis for biomedical applications are private, making the result comparison impossible (Orozco-Arroyave et al. 2015; Saenz-Lechon et al. 2006). To the best of our knowledge, there are several publicly available databases, which are shown in Table 1.2 along with their basic statistical information.

The MEEI database is commercially available, which contains English voices from 53 healthy and 657 pathological speakers. Each sample consists of the first part of the Rainbow passage and the sustained vowel/a/. All voices were sampled with 16-bit resolution. The sampling rate of normal samples was 50 kHz, while that of pathological voices was 25 kHz or 50 kHz. MEEI has been a benchmark for decades, on which the highest accuracy of detecting pathological voice reaches $100.0 \pm 0.0\%$ (Mekyska et al. 2015). However, it should be emphasized that the voices of patients and healthy subjects in MEEI were collected in two different environments and with different sampling rates. These differences may lead to biased accuracy in the detection of pathological voice. It was stated in Mekyska et al. (2015) that MEEI should no longer be used as a benchmark. More discussions on the MEEI database can be found in Saenz-Lechon et al. (2006).

The Saarbruecken Voice Database (SVD) database recorded by the Institute of Phonetics of Saarland University in Germany is freely available (Barry and Putzer 2012). All voices in SVD were sampled at 50 kHz with 16-bit resolution in the same

Table 1.2 Publicly available databases for computerized voice analysis

Dataset	Sample	Language	Pathologies	Contents
MEEI (Elemetrics 1994)	53 + 657	English	Various types	Audios: Vowels and sentences
SVD (Barry and Putzer 2012)	650 + 1320	Germany	71 types	Audios: Vowels and sentences
PdA (Mekyska et al. 2015)	239 + 200	Spanish	Various types	Audios: vowels
PDS (Little 2008)	8 + 23	English	PD only	Features: 22-dimensional
PTDS (Tsanas and Little 2009)	0 + 42	English	PD only	Features: 16-dimensional

The sample column is shown as No. of normal speakers + No. of pathological speakers. The last database is for monitoring only environment. There are more than 2000 speakers in SVD, where the pathological ones are from 71 different diseases. The recordings for each speaker include vowels / a/, /i/, and/u/ produced at normal, high, low, and low-high-low pitch, together with a sentence in German "Guten Morgen, wie geht es Ihnen?" ("Good morning, how are you?"). This database is quite new, on which few studies have been conducted (Al-nasheri et al. 2017b; Muhammad et al. 2017).

Pathological voices in the Principe de Asturias (PdA) database, which is freely available for research purposes, were recorded from patients with organic diseases (Mekyska et al. 2015). The PdA database consists of voices from 239 healthy and 200 pathological speakers. Each sample contains a sustained Spanish vowel /a/, sampled at 25 kHz with 16-bit resolution. Experiments in Mekyska et al. (2015) demonstrated that it was challenging to detect pathological voices on PdA database, on which large scope of improvements may be made in the future.

The MEEI, SVD, and PdA databases all contain pathological voices of several diseases. The Parkinson's dataset (PDS) (Little 2008) and Parkinson's telemonitoring dataset (PTDS) (Tsanas and Little 2009) in the UCI Machine Learning Repository (freely available), however, are uniquely for Parkinson's disease. Besides, instead of voice signals, PDS and PTDS are composed of biomedical voice measurements extracted from sustained vowels /a/ for the detection and monitoring of PD, respectively. In PDS, 16-dimensional features are extracted for each of the 195 voice recordings from 23 patients with PD and 8 healthy controls. PTDS contains 16-dimensional measurements for each of the 5875 voice recordings collected from 42 patients with early stage PD. Even though only features rather than voice are publicly available in the PDS and PTDS, classification and regression experiments can be performed (Hariharan et al. 2014; Chen et al. 2013).

1.2.3.2 Feature Extraction

Various kinds of features are used in computerized voice analysis. For example, the Multi-Dimensional Voice Program (MDVP) Elemetrics (2012), which is a typical software for pathological voice analysis, provides 33 features for each recording. Studies (Tsanas et al. 2011; Orozco-Arroyave et al. 2015; Mekyska et al. 2015; Alonso et al. 2001; Gelzinis et al. 2008) gave more features. In this section, important features in computerized voice analysis are categorized, as illustrated in Table 1.3. Note that if the features listed in Table 1.3 in sequence are from the same reference, only the last one is marked with the associated reference in order to save space. In addition, the features listed here are by no means exhaustive since our aim is for categorization.

First, based on the domain where features are extracted, there are three major classes: time domain, frequency domain, and wavelet domain.

- Time domain: short-time energy (STE) (measures the strength of signal and a low STD may indicate hypophonia) and zero-crossing rate (ZCR) (describes the times that a voice waveform crosses the zero axes within a given time) are typical

Table 1.3 Categorization of features in computerized voice analysis. If the listed features in sequence are from the same reference, only the last one is marked with the associated reference

Category	Sub-category	Typical features
Domain	Time domain	STE, ZCR (Mekyska et al. 2015), RAP, DVB, DUV, NVB, NUS (Elemetrics 2012)
	Frequency domain	HNR (Tsanas 2012), NHR (Elemetrics 2012), MFCC (Tsanas 2012), formants (Muhammad et al. 2011), spectrum decomposition (Markaki and Stylianou 2011), modulation spectra (Mekyska et al. 2015).
	Wavelet domain	PP (Scalassara et al. 2009), RMS and jitter of reconstructed wavelet components (Fonseca and Pereira 2009)
Observations	Stability	Jitter, shimmer (Elemetrics 2012), RPDE (Tsanas 2012)
	Noise level	NHR, NNE, VTI, SPI (Elemetrics 2012)
Vocal systems	Vocal folds	GNE, GQopen, GQclosed (Tsanas 2012), IDP (Muhammad et al. 2017)
	Vocal tract	F1, F2, F3, B1, B2, B3 (Mekyska et al. 2015)
Nonlinear theory	Nonlinear dynamic	CD, FD, LZC, HE, SHE, CE, AE, SE, LLE (Mekyska et al. 2015)
	EMD	SNR defined with IMFs (Tsanas et al. 2011)
	High-order spectrum	BII, HFEB, LFEB, BMII, BPII (Alonso et al. 2001)

features to assess the quality of voice (Mekyska et al. 2015). Features in MDVP (Elemetrics 2012) calculated in time domain include relative average perturbation (RAP), degree of voice breaks (DVB), degree of voiceless (DUV), number of voice breaks (NVB), and number of unvoiced segments (NUS).

- Frequency domain: many features are based on the voice spectrum (features based on short-time Fourier transform (STFT) also fall into this category). Some examples are harmonics to noise ratio (HNR) (a low HNR may imply breathiness or hoarseness) (Tsanas 2012), noise to harmonic ratio (NHR) (Elemetrics 2012), Mel frequency cepstral coefficients (MFCC) and its derivatives (Tsanas 2012), formants (Muhammad et al. 2011), spectrum based decomposition (Markaki and Stylianou 2011; Gomez et al. 2005), mean power in different frequency bands (Fraile et al. 2013), and the features based on modulation spectra Mekyska et al. 2015). In particular, it was experimentally proved that the power level in high frequency bands (above 5300 Hz) was significantly different for normal and pathological voices (Fraile et al. 2013).
- Wavelet domain: predictive power (PP) proposed in Scalassara et al. 2009) was calculated based on the wavelet decomposition. In Fonseca and Pereira (2009), statistics of reconstructed discrete wavelet components were used as features to detect pathological voices and to identify pathology. Study in Mahbub and Shahnaz (2015) put forward to use normalized energy contents of the discrete wavelet transform (DWT) coefficients for the detection of voice disorders.

Second, based on the intuitive observations of pathological voice, there exist two groups of features describing the stability and noise level, respectively.

- Stability: in MDVP (Elemetrics 2012), parameter describing the fundamental frequency variability in time (named as jitter) and its variants are used to evaluate the frequency perturbation of voice; parameter measuring the variability of amplitude in time (namely shimmer) and its variants are to assess the intensity perturbation. The recurrence probability density entropy feature (RPDE) describes the dispersion level of pitch period in a sustained vowel (Tsanas 2012). It was demonstrated that features describing stability were most suitable to assess three pathologies: PD, laryngeal pathologies (LP), and CLP (Orozco-Arroyave et al. 2015).
- Noise level: noise measurements describe the degree of voice hoarseness, breathiness, and hypernasality. Harmonics to noise ratio (HNR), normalized noise energy (NNE), voice turbulence index (VTI), and soft phonation index (SPI) are some noise measurements in MDVP (Elemetrics 2012). Readers may refer Orozco-Arroyave et al. (2015) and (Mekyska et al. 2015) for more details. Even though these measures may be effective for high-quality voice, it was demonstrated in Moran et al. (2006) that HNR measures are not suitable for remote pathological/normal identification.

Third, based on the mechanism of voice production, there are two classes of features describing the functioning of vocal folds and vocal tract, respectively.

- Vocal folds: Glottal-to-noise excitation ratio (GNE) (Tsanas 2012), glottal quotients (GQopen and GQclosed) (Tsanas 2012), and interlaced derivative pattern (IDP) (Muhammad et al. 2017) are features extracted from the estimated glottal source excitation. An experiment in Muhammad et al. (2017) showed that using glottal waveform rather than the input voice was beneficial to detect pathology in vocal folds.
- Vocal tract: vocal tract can be characterized by formants. In Mekyska et al. (Mekyska et al. 2015), frequencies of the first three formants F1, F2, F3 and their bandwidths B1, B2, B3 were used to describe the tongue movement in pathological voice. Formants related features in Orozco-Arroyave et al. (2015) displayed high discriminating power in detecting hypernasality, which is a common symptom for patients with CLP.

Finally, extracted features can also be grouped based on the assumptions in voice modeling. Traditionally, vocal tract is presumed as linear in the production of voice and thus there is no existence of nonlinearity in the voice signal. However, it has been proved that vocal tract is nonlinear in practice (Teager and Teager 1990). Hence, several nonlinear approaches are introduced to extract features.

- Nonlinear dynamic: nonlinear dynamic analysis is suitable to characterize pathological voice, especially to voices with subharmonics and chaos where traditional techniques may fail (Mekyska et al. 2015). Representative features based on nonlinear dynamic analysis include correlation dimension (CD), fractal dimension (FD), Lempel–Ziv complexity (LZC), Hurst exponent (HE), Shannon entropy (SHE), correlation entropy (CE), approximate entropy (AE), sample entropy (SE), and largest Lyapunov exponent (LLE). Most of these features can be extracted by the TISEAN software (Hegger et al. 1999). More details of features in the category of nonlinear dynamic can be found in the following works (Henriquez et al. 2009; Lopez-de Ipina et al. 2013; Orozco-Arroyave et al. 2015; Mekyska et al. 2015).

- Empirical mode decomposition (EMD): EMD is a nonlinear tool that decomposes a nonlinear signal into elementary components called intrinsic mode functions (IMF). Tsanas et al. (2011) considered the first few IMFs as noise in voice and the remaining IMFs as actual useful information. Then features quantifying the ratio of signal energy to noise energy were defined. See details in Tsanas et al. (2011).
- High-order spectrum: comparing with pathological voice, healthy voice shows a greater presence of quadratic phase coupling (Alonso et al. 2001), which can be characterized by bispectrum analysis. A detection rate of 98.3% was reached on a private database with the bispectrum based features, including bicoherence index interference (BII), high frequency energy of one-dimensional bicoherence (HFEB), low frequency energy of one-dimensional bicoherence (LFEB), bispectrum module interference index (BMII), and bispectrum phase interference index (BPII).

1.2.3.3 Classification and Regression

In machine learning, a common modeling task is to predict responses for new observations using the model learned from historical data whose responses are known. When the responses are discrete labels, it will be a classification problem. Otherwise, regression algorithms are utilized to predict continuous values. In terms of computerized voice analysis, classification and regression algorithms are needed for pathology detection (classification) and monitoring, as presented in Table 1.4.

- Pathology detection and identification: Support vector machine (SVM) is the most frequently used classifier (Dibazar et al. 2002; Markaki and Stylianou 2009, 2011; Tsanas et al. 2012; Little et al. 2009; Arjmandi and Pooyan 2012; Vikram and Umarani 2013; Saeedi et al. 2011; Arjmandi et al. 2011; Alsulaiman 2014; Cavalcanti et al. 2010; Zhou et al. 2012; Saeedi and Almasganj 2013; Orozco-Arroyave et al. 2011, 2015; Al-nasheri et al. 2017a, b; Muhammad et al. 2017; Fonseca and Pereira 2009; Hariharan et al. 2014; Chen et al. 2013; Gelzinis et al.

Table 1.4 Classification and regression methods used in computerized voice analysis

Task	Method
Pathology detection	SVM (Dibazar et al. 2002), RF (Tsanas et al. 2012), NN (Henriquez et al. 2009), HMM (Saudi et al. 2012), GMM (Godino-Llorente et al. 2006), Bayesian classifier (Castellanos et al. 2006)
Severity prediction	LS (Tsanas et al. 2010), IRLS (Tsanas et al. 2010), LASSO (Tsanas et al. 2010), ISVR (Nilashi et al. 2018), CART (Tsanas et al. 2010), RF (Tsanas et al. 2011), ELM (Wang et al. 2016), SVM (Wang et al. 2016), CDT (Le et al. 2014), LR (Le et al. 2014), NB (Le et al. 2014)

2008), especially with the radial basis function kernel (RBF). Notice that SVM is a common choice for both binary (pathological detection) and multi-class classification problem (pathology type identification) (Markaki and Stylianou 2009, 2011; Alsulaiman 2014; Cavalcanti et al. 2010; Saeedi and Almasganj 2013; Al-nasheri et al. 2017b; Muhammad et al. 2017; Fonseca and Pereira 2009; Gelzinis et al. 2008). Other classifiers used include random forest (RF) (Tsanas et al. 2012; Arora et al. 2015; Mekyska et al. 2015), neural network (NN) (Henríquez et al. 2009; Lopez-de Ipina et al. 2013; Akbari and Arjmandi 2014; Saenz-Lechon et al. 2006; Muhammad et al. 2011; Alonso et al. 2001), hidden Markov model (HMM) (Saudi et al. 2012; Jothilakshmi 2014; Alsulaiman 2014), Gaussian mixture model (GMM) (Godino-Llorente et al. 2006; Jothilakshmi 2014; Alsulaiman 2014), k-nearest neighbor (KNN) (Arjmandi and Pooyan 2012; Hadjitodorov and Mitev 2002; Arjmandi et al. 2011; Chen et al. 2013; Gelzinis et al. 2008), and Bayesian classifier (Castellanos et al. 2006). The performance of each classifier depends on the data for classification. For instance, RF gave higher accuracy rates than SVM (with a RBF kernel) on two out of three databases in Mekyska et al. (2015), but reached lower accuracy in Tsanas et al. (2012) and Tsanas et al. (2011). Nevertheless, extensive experiments in Fernandez-Delgado et al. (2014) showed that RF and SVM were most likely to give the best performances in many classification problems.

- Monitoring: comparing with detection, monitoring by computerized voice analysis is less studied. Disease severity can be assessed with either a classifier or a regression algorithm. Regarding regression algorithms, it was shown in Tsanas et al. (2010) that CART (classification and regression tree) had lower mean absolute error than least squares (LS), iteratively reweighted least squares (IRLS), and least absolute shrinkage and selection operator (LASSO). Furthermore, experiments in Tsanas et al. (2011) proved that CART was inferior to RF in predicting the symptom severity of PD. Another regression algorithm used to predict the severity of PD was Incremental Support Vector Regression (ISVR) (Nilashi et al. 2018). On the other hand, severity prediction problem can be solved in a classification mode (Wang et al. 2016; Le et al. 2014). In Wang et al. (2016), the quality of pathological voice was rated on a 4-point scale: normal, slight, moderate, and severe dysphonia, where extreme learning machine (ELM) offered better performances than SVM. The treatment of aphasia was assessed in Le et al. (2014) with six classifiers (C4.5 decision tree (CDT), logistic regression (LR), naive Bayes (NB), RF, and SVM), where RF showed the highest accuracy.

1.2.3.4 Deep Learning Based Computerized Voice Analysis

In the traditional pattern recognition paradigm, feature extraction and classification (regression) steps are performed separately, as shown in Sects. 1.2.3.2 and 1.2.3.3. However, the recent popular deep learning algorithms often learn the complex mapping function between (simply preprocessed) input signals and the outputs (labels) directly by constructing a neural networks of multiple hidden layers, which has been shown great success in the field of image recognition (Donahue et al. 2014), speaker recognition (Richardson et al. 2015), musical information retrieval (Vaizman et al. 2014), and ECG (electrocardiogram) based classification (Al Rahhal et al. 2016). Therefore, researchers also introduce this technique into computerized voice analysis for biomedical application. In Frid et al. (2016), it was proposed to split a continuous speech into overlapping frames and regard the datapoints of each frame as the input to a Convolutional Neural Network (CNN). Finally, a majority voting scheme was used to fuse the CNN decision of all segmented frames. Study in Harar et al. (2017) also used the raw audio signal as input to a deep neural networks (DNN). In Vasquez et al. (2017) and Zhang et al. (2018), however, the time-frequency representations of voice was input into a CNN for PD detection. In addition, deep neural network can also be regarded as a classifier, in which hand-crafted features are the input of the network as in Zhang et al. (2017) and Fang et al. (2018).

As pointed out in Sect. 1.2.4, small sample size is quite common in computerized voice analysis and it poses a great challenge, especially when deep learning technique is used, which often has large amounts of parameters to be learned. To deal with this issue, authors in Alhussein and Muhammad (2018) proposed to detect voice pathology by using transfer learning on two robust CNN models. In detail, the CNN models were pretrained on a very large numbers of images, and the weights of the pretrained network were fine-tuned using the training samples of the voice pathology database.

1.2.3.5 State-of-the-Art Result on the Publicly Available Dataset

The former parts in this section present the developments of each step in computerized voice analysis. Finally, we show the state-of-the-art results on publicly available database. As seen in Table 1.5, computerized voice analysis is promising for disease detection and monitoring, especially on database like MEEI and PDS. However, there are still challenges to put computerized voice analysis into clinical use, as we will discuss in the next section.

1.2.4 Open Challenges in Computerized Voice Analysis

There are still several major open challenges to be handled before putting the computerized voice analysis into clinical use. In this section, the existing challenges are discussed in terms of data level and algorithm level. Eventually, we attempt to propose several suggestions on the future research directions. The challenges and future directions are summarized in Fig. 1.2, with "(C)" representing challenges and "(D)" denoting the directions.

Table 1.5 State-of-the-art results on publicly available database in Table 1.2

Database	Task	Important features	Classifier (regression)	Performance
MEEI (Elemetrics 1994)	Detect PV	Modulation spectra, etc.	RF	Acc = 100.0% (Mekyska et al. 2015)
SVD (Barry and Putzer 2012)	Detect PV	MFCC, HNR, GNE, etc.	GMM	Acc = 79.4% (Martınez et al. 2012)
PdA (Mekyska et al. 2015)	Detect PV	Modulation spectra, etc.	RF	Acc = 82.1% (Mekyska et al. 2015)
PDS (Little 2008)	Detect PD	Jitter, shimmer, RPDE, DFA, etc.	SVM	Acc = 98.5% (Tsanas 2012)
PTDS (Tsanas and Little 2009)	Predict PD severity	Jitter, shimmer, RPDE, DFA, PPE, etc.	ISVR	MAE = 0.4967 (Nilashi et al. 2018)

"PV" and "Acc" in this table represent pathological voice and classification accuracy, respectively

1.2.4.1   Data Level Challenges

Dataset with both pathological and normal voice are needed in developing a practical computerized voice analysis system, on which the model as well as the parameters in the system can be optimized. However, it is not trivial to prepare such database. The possible challenges are discussed as follows.

- Small sample size, especially for a rare disease. Unlike machine learning task like speaker and speech recognition, sample size in computerized voice analysis can be rather small where the intrinsic characteristics of voices for a certain disease cannot be well represented and overfitting could occur (Wasikowski and Chen 2010). Since it is often difficult to increase the sample size, researchers tend to apply carefully designed algorithms to handle this issue, as discussed in Sect. 1.2.4.2.
- Biased sample size results in imbalance classification. More discussion on this issue is presented in Sect. 1.2.4.2.
- There are few evidenced guidelines on recording voice for computerized voice analysis. The effects of the environment SNR (signal-to-noise ratio), noise type, sampling parameters (sampling rate and quantization bits), and the required phonation text (such as sustained vowels and continuous sentences) on computerized voice analysis are rarely investigated. Specially, the effect of noise level and type determine whether computerized voice analysis can be widely used and thus study similar to Poorjam et al. (2017) is highly demanded.
- Even though there have been several published databases containing pathological and normal voices, e.g., MEEI (Elemetrics 1994) and SVD (Barry and Putzer 2012), it can be problematic to merge them to form a bigger database since the recording environment (SNR and the possible noise type), hardware, languages, and the required texts are quite different from each other (Al-nasheri et al. 2017a).

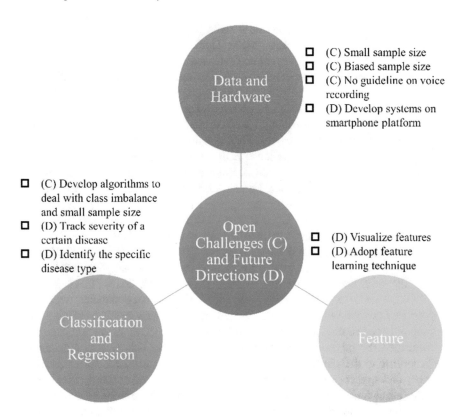

Fig. 1.2 Open challenges and future directions of computerized voice analysis

1.2.4.2 Algorithm Level Challenges

Algorithms in computerized voice analysis are used to extract features and to build models for diagnosis (monitoring). In this section, we mainly discuss the challenges in building model for diagnosis.

- As discussed in Sect. 1.2.4.1, small sample size is one major obstacle. Besides, the dimension of extracted features is often high so that the characteristics of data can be described fully. For instance, the feature dimension in Tsanas et al. (2012) is 318. Hence, the ill-posed challenge of high dimensional low sample size (HDLSS) arises, where an outlier point in the dataset can affect the performance of diagnosis severely. Studies to deal with this problem can generally be divided into two categories, with one concerning dimension reduction (Qiu et al. 2014; Dernoncourt et al. 2014) and the other devising robust and regularized classification algorithms (Gunduz and Fokoue 2015). In Zhang and Lin (2013), Zhang and Lin proposed that classifiers to deal with HDLSS issue should satisfy six properties, including predictability, consistency, generality, stability, robustness, and sparsity. Developing classifiers satisfying these demands is challenging. Studies in Yata and Aoshima (2012), Dutta and Ghosh (2016) and Bolivar-Cime and Marron (2013) present more discussion on the HDLSS problem.

- Class imbalance is a common challenge in many medical diagnosis applications. In computerized voice analysis, class imbalance refers to the occasion that the number of patients with a certain disease is far less than the number of healthy subjects. The skewed distribution leads to performance loss for many machine learning algorithms and the resulting classifiers are often biased toward the majority class, which misdiagnose patients as being healthy. In addition, six types of data characteristics even complicate the class imbalance classification problem as discussed in Lopez, Fernandez, Garcia, Palade, and Herrera (Lopez et al. 2013): small disjuncts, density lack in the training data, overlapping between classes, presence of noisy data, borderline instances, and the dataset shift between training and test distributions. Researchers have proposed intense work to solve the problem of class imbalance (He et al. 2008; Ting 2000; Xu et al. 2016), which can be divided into three classes: data sampling, algorithmic modification, and cost-sensitive learning (Lopez et al. 2013). In Galar et al. (2012), ensembles based method was added into the categorization, which was regarded as more versatile without dependence of the base classifier. Moreover, to improve the classification further, study in Napierala and Stefanowski (2016) first identified the minority class examples in a concrete dataset into four classes according to their influence on the classification performance: safe, borderline, rare, and outliers (Napierala and Stefanowski 2016). The interested reader is referred to find more suggestions on the solutions to class-imbalance problem in (Lopez et al. 2013; Galar et al. 2012; Napierala and Stefanowski 2016; Krawczyk 2016; Prati et al. 2015; Beyan and Fisher 2015).

1.2.5   Future Directions in Computerized Voice Analysis

Some possible future research directions in computerized voice analysis are listed.

- Aside from the binary classification in detecting pathological voice, there are demands to implement multi-class classification to identify the specific pathology type. However, previous research on identifying disease type (Markaki and Stylianou 2009, 2011; Arjmandi and Pooyan 2012; Jothilakshmi 2014; Alsulaiman 2014; Cavalcanti et al. 2010) are much less than those aiming only to discriminate pathological voice from the normal one (Dibazar et al. 2002; Godino-Llorente et al. 2006; Henrıquez et al. 2009; Hadjitodorov and Mitev 2002; Vikram and Umarani 2013; Boyanov and Hadjitodorov 1997; Saeedi et al. 2011; Arjmandi et al. 2011). In the future, diagnosis with computerized voice analysis should pay more attention to identifying the pathology type.
- Visualize the extracted features. In the current clinical setting, it is desirable to develop an interactive system to combine computerized features with doctors' experience-based diagnosis, in which feature visualization is needed. When more

features are developed for diagnosis and monitoring in modern acoustical analysis, dimension reduction and visualization techniques should be adopted in order to obtain insights into pathological voices (Goddard et al. 2009).

- Predict the severity of a certain disease. While most studies focus on screening out diseases (either a single type or several types together) by voice analysis (Dibazar et al. 2002; Markaki and Stylianou 2009, 2011; Tsanas et al. 2011, 2012; Little et al. 2009; Arjmandi and Pooyan 2012; Vikram and Umarani 2013; Saeedi et al. 2011; Arjmandi et al. 2011; Alsulaiman 2014; Cavalcanti et al. 2010; Zhou et al. 2012; Saeedi and Almasganj 2013; Orozco-Arroyave et al. 2011, 2015; Al-nasheri et al. 2017a, b; Muhammad et al. 2011, 2017; Fonseca and Pereira 2009; Hariharan et al. 2014; Chen et al. 2013; Gelzinis et al. 2008; Arora et al. 2015; Mekyska et al. 2015; Henrıquez et al. 2009; Lopez-de Ipina et al. 2013; Akbari and Arjmandi 2014; Saenz-Lechon et al. 2006; Alonso et al. 2001; Saudi et al. 2012; Jothilakshmi 2014; Godino-Llorente et al. 2006; Hadjitodorov and Mitev 2002; Castellanos et al. 2006; Fernandez-Delgado et al. 2014), it is necessary to track the progression of disease, especially for a chronic one (Tsanas et al. 2010, 2011; Wang et al. 2016; Le et al. 2014; Nilashi et al. 2018). With severity prediction algorithm, it can also help to assess the effectiveness of a given treatment.
- Develop systems in smartphone platform. With increasing computing capacities and popularity of smartphone, it is interesting to assess the feasibility of applying the computerized voice analysis on smartphone (Rusz et al. 2018; Manfredi et al. 2017), which is more affordable and convenient for consumers.
- Remote computerized voice analysis. Remote voice analysis is meaningful since it can not only provide therapy for populations in remote regions, but also ensure the participation of patients, who may otherwise discontinue their treatment prematurely (Moran et al. 2006). To transmit voice over long distances (via telephone network or Internet), the quality of voice is often degraded due to compression, band limiting, channel filtering, and additive noise. Even though there has been some research (Moran et al. 2006; Fraile et al. 2009; Kaleem et al. 2011; Reilly et al. 2004) studying the impact of these quality-degrading factors on the performance of voice based disease detection and monitoring, the performance of remote voice analysis needs to be improved further.
- In terms of algorithms in computerized voice analysis, we point out that a majority of widely used features are hand-crafted. The success of feature learning in the field of image recognition (Donahue et al. 2014), speaker recognition (Richardson et al. 2015), musical information retrieval (Vaizman et al. 2014), and ECG (electrocardiogram) based classification (Al Rahhal et al. 2016) motivates us to investigate the performance of learned features in computerized voice analysis.

1.2.6 Summary

The advantages of computerized technologies give rise to computerized voice analysis. In this section, research on voice analysis in biomedical applications are reviewed to reemphasize the biomedical value of voice. Firstly, a comprehensive literature review is carried out, revealing that many diseases show signs in voice. In addition, based on the voice production mechanism, we categorize the diseases affecting voice into three classes. The categories are nerve system diseases, respiratory system diseases, and diseases in vocal folds and vocal tract. Secondly, the three steps in computerized voice analysis, which are voice recording, feature extraction, and classification (regression), are reviewed separately. Finally, the potential challenges to be addressed in computerized voice analysis are discussed in data level and algorithm level. Besides, we also give some suggestions concerning future research directions.

Voice is often used for speaker and speech recognition. Now biomedical value of voice is reemphasized, forming the third main application of voice. We hope this work may contribute to the further development of computerized voice analysis in the biomedical field.

References

Akbari, A., & Arjmandi, M. K. (2014). An efficient voice pathology classification scheme based on applying multi-layer linear discriminant analysis to wavelet packet-based features. *Biomed. Signal Process. Control*, 10, 209–223.

Al-nasheri, A., Muhammad, G., Alsulaiman, M., & Ali, Z. (2017a). Investigation of voice pathology detection and classification on different frequency regions using correlation functions. *J. Voice*, 31, 3–15.

Al-nasheri, A., Muhammad, G., Alsulaiman, M., Ali, Z., Mesallam, T. A., Farahat, M., Malki, K. H., & Bencherif, M. A. (2017b). An investigation of multidimensional voice program parameters in three different databases for voice pathology detection and classification. *J. Voice*, 31, 113.e9–113.e18.

Al Rahhal, M. M., Bazi, Y., AlHichri, H., Alajlan, N., Melgani, F., & Yager, R. R. (2016). Deep learning approach for active classification of electrocardiogram signals. *Inf. Sci.*, 345, 340–354.

Alhussein, M., & Muhammad, G. (2018). Voice pathology detection using deep learning on mobile healthcare framework. *IEEE Access*, (pp. 1–1).

Alonso, J. B., De Leon, J., Alonso, I., & Ferrer, M. A. (2001). Automatic detection of pathologies in the voice by hos based parameters. *EURASIP J. Appl. Signal Process.*, 4, 275–284.

Alsulaiman, M. (2014). Voice pathology assessment systems for dysphonic patients: Detection, classification, and speech recognition. *IETE J. Res.*, 60, 156–167.

Arjmandi, M. K., & Pooyan, M. (2012). An optimum algorithm in pathological voice quality assessment using wavelet-packet-based features, linear discriminant analysis and support vector machine. *Biomed. Signal Process. Control*, 7, 3–19.

Arjmandi, M. K., Pooyan, M., Mikaili, M., Vali, M., & Moqarehzadeh, A. (2011). Identification of voice disorders using long-time features and support vector machine with different feature reduction methods. *J. Voice*, 25, e275–e289.

Arora, S., Venkataraman, V., Zhan, A., Donohue, S., Biglan, K., Dorsey, E., & Little, M. (2015). Detecting and monitoring the symptoms of Parkinson's disease using smartphones: a pilot study. *Parkinsonism Relat. Disord.*, 21, 650–653.

Atal, B. S. (1972). Automatic speaker recognition based on pitch contours. *J. Acoust. Soc. Am.*, 52 (6B), 1687-1697.

Barry, W. J., and Putzer, M. (2012). Saarbrucken voice database, institute of phonetics. Available at http://www.stimmdatenbank.coli.uni-saarland.de/.

Benba, A. (2016). A review of the assessment methods of voice disorders in the context of Parkinson's disease. *J. Telecommun. Electron. Comput. Eng.*, 8, 103–112.

Beyan, C., & Fisher, R. (2015). Classifying imbalanced data sets using similarity based hierarchical decomposition. *Pattern Recognit.*, 48, 1653–1672.

Bolivar-Cime, A., & Marron, J. (2013). Comparison of binary discrimination methods for high dimension low sample size data. *J. Multivariate Anal.*, 115, 108–121.

Boyanov, B., & Hadjitodorov, S. (1997). Acoustic analysis of pathological voices: a voice analysis system for the screening of laryngeal diseases. *IEEE Eng. Med. Biol. Mag.*, 16, 74–82.

Brauers, A., Kellner, A., Lanfermann, G., & Te, V. J. (2006). Automated speech disorder detection method and apparatus.

Campisi, P., Tewfik, T. L., Pelland-Blais, E., Husein, M., & Sadeghi, N. (2000). Multidimensional voice program analysis in children with vocal cord nodules. J. *Otolaryngol. Head Neck Surg.*, 29, 302.

Castellanos, G., Daza, G., Sanchez, L., Castrillon, O., & Suarez, J. (2006). Acoustic speech analysis for hypernasality detection in children. *In Annu. Int. Conf. IEEE Eng. Med. Biol. Soc.* (pp. 5507–5510).

Cavalcanti, N., Silva, S., Bresolin, A., Bezerra, H., & Guerreiro, A. (2010). Comparative analysis between wavelets for the identification of pathological voices. *Prog. Pattern Recognit., Image Anal., Comput. Vision, Appl.*, (pp. 236–243).

Chen, H.-L., Huang, C.-C., Yu, X.-G., Xu, X., Sun, X., Wang, G., & Wang, S.-J. (2013). An efficient diagnosis system for detection of Parkinson's disease using fuzzy k-nearest neighbor approach. Expert Syst. Appl., 40, 263–271.

David, A. L. J. (2010). Stochastic characterization of nonlinear dynamics for the automatic evaluation of voice quality. Ph.D. thesis Dept. Circuits Syst., Universidad Politecnica de Madrid, Madrid, ES.

De Bruijn, M. J., Ten Bosch, L., Kuik, D. J., Quene, H., Langendijk, J. A., Leemans, C. R., & Verdonck-de Leeuw, I. M. (2009). Objective acoustic phonetic speech analysis in patients treated for oral or oropharyngeal cancer. *Folia. Phoniatr. Logop.*, 61, 180–187.

Dernoncourt, D., Hanczar, B., & Zucker, J.-D. (2014). Analysis of feature selection stability on high dimension and small sample data. *Comput. Stat. Data Anal.*, 71, 681–693.

Dibazar, A. A., Narayanan, S., & Berger, T. W. (2002). Feature analysis for automatic detection of pathological speech. *In Proc. 2nd Joint EMBS-BMES Conf. Ann. Int. Conf. Eng. Med Biol. Soc. Ann. Fall Meet. Biomed. Eng. Soc.* (pp. 182–183).

Donahue, J., Jia, Y., Vinyals, O., Hoffman, J., Zhang, N., Tzeng, E., & Darrell, T. (2014). Decaf: A deep convolutional activation feature for generic visual recognition. *In Proc. Int. Conf. Mach. Learn.* (pp. 647–655).

Dutta, S., & Ghosh, A. K. (2016). On some transformations of high dimension, low sample size data for nearest neighbor classification. *Mach. Learn.*, 102, 57–83.

Elemetrics, K. (1994). Voice disorders database, version. 1.03 [CD-ROM].

Elemetrics, K. (2012). Multi-dimensional voice program (MDVP) [computer program].

Fang, S.-H., Tsao, Y., Hsiao, M.-J., Chen, J.-Y., Lai, Y.-H., Lin, F.-C., & Wang, C.-T. (2018). Detection of pathological voice using cepstrum vectors: A deep learning approach. *J. Voice*.

Fernandez-Delgado, M., Cernadas, E., Barro, S., & Amorim, D. (2014). Do we need hundreds of classifiers to solve real world classification problems. *J. Mach. Learn. Res.*, 15, 3133–3181.

Fonseca, E. S., & Pereira, J. C. (2009). Normal versus pathological voice signals. *IEEE Eng. Med. Biol. Mag.*, 28.

Fraile, R., Godino-Llorente, J. I., Saenz-Lechon, N., Osma-Ruiz, V., & Gutierrez-Arriola, J. M. (2013). Characterization of dysphonic voices by means of a filterbank-based spectral analysis: sustained vowels and running speech. *J. Voice*, 27, 11–23.

Fraile, R., Saenz-Lechon, N., Godino-Llorente, J. I., Osma-Ruiz, V., & Fredouille, C. (2009). Mfcc-based remote pathology detection on speech transmitted through the telephone channel - impact of linear distortions: Band limitation, frequency response and noise. In *Proc. Biosignals* (pp. 41–48).

Frid, A., Kantor, A., Svechin, D., & Manevitz, L. M. (2016). Diagnosis of Parkinson's disease from continuous speech using deep convolutional networks without manual selection of features. In *2016 IEEE Int. Conf. Sci. Electr. Eng.* (pp. 1–4).

Galar, M., Fernandez, A., Barrenechea, E., Bustince, H., & Herrera, F. (2012). A review on ensembles for the class imbalance problem: bagging-, boosting-, and hybrid-based approaches. *IEEE Trans. Syst. Man Cybern. Part C Appl. Rev.*, 42, 463–484.

Garcia, N., Orozco-Arroyave, J. R., D'Haro, L., Dehak, N., & Garcia, E. N. (2017). Evaluation of the neurological state of people with Parkinson's disease using i-vectors. In *Proc. Interspeech* (pp. 299–303).

Gelzinis, A., Verikas, A., & Bacauskiene, M. (2008). Automated speech analysis applied to laryngeal disease categorization. *Comput. Methods Programs Biomed.*, 91, 36–47.

Goddard, J., Schlotthauer, G., Torres, M., & Rufiner, H. (2009). Dimensionality reduction for visualization of normal and pathological speech data. *Biomed. Signal Process. Control*, 4, 194–201.

Godino-Llorente, J. I., Gomez-Vilda, P., & Blanco-Velasco, M. (2006). Dimensionality reduction of a pathological voice quality assessment system based on Gaussian mixture models and short-term cepstral parameters. *IEEE Trans. Biomed. Eng.*, 53, 1943–1953.

Gomez, P., Dıaz, F., Alvarez, A., Murphy, K., Lazaro, C., Martınez, R., & Rodellar, V. (2005). Principal component analysis of spectral perturbation parameters for voice pathology detection. In *Proc. 18th IEEE Symp. Computer Based Med. Syst.* (pp. 41–46).

Graves, A., Mohamed, A. R., & Hinton, G. (2013). Speech recognition with deep recurrent neural networks. *IEEE Int. Conf. Acoust.*

Gunduz, N., & Fokoue, E. (2015). Robust classification of high dimension low sample size data. Available at https://arxiv.org/abs/1501.00592.

Hadjitodorov, S., & Mitev, P. (2002). A computer system for acoustic analysis of pathological voices and laryngeal diseases screening. *Med. Eng. Phys.*, 24, 419–429.

Hamdan, A.-L., Medawar, W., Younes, A., Bikhazi, H., & Fuleihan, N. (2005). The effect of hemodialysis on voice: an acoustic analysis. *J. Voice*, 19, 290–295.

Harar, P., Alonso-Hernandezy, J. B., Mekyska, J., Galaz, Z., Burget, R., & Smekal, Z. (2017). Voice pathology detection using deep learning: a preliminary study. In *Int. Conf. Workshop on Bioinspired Intell.* (pp. 1–4).

Harel, B., Cannizzaro, M., & Snyder, P. J. (2004). Variability in fundamental frequency during speech in prodromal and incipient Parkinson's disease: A longitudinal case study. *Brain. Cogn.*, 56, 24–29.

Hariharan, M., Polat, K., & Sindhu, R. (2014). A new hybrid intelligent system for accurate detection of Parkinson's disease. *Comput. Methods Programs Biomed.*, 113, 904–913.

He, H., Bai, Y., Garcia, E. A., & Li, S. (2008). ADASYN: Adaptive synthetic sampling approach for imbalanced learning. In *IEEE Int. Joint Conf. Neural Netw.* (pp. 1322–1328).

Hegger, R., Kantz, H., & Schreiber, T. (1999). Practical implementation of nonlinear time series methods: The TISEAN package. *Chaos*, 9, 413–435.

Henrıquez, P., Alonso, J. B., Ferrer, M. A., Travieso, C. M., Godino-Llorente, J. I., & Dıaz-de Marıa, F. (2009). Characterization of healthy and pathological voice through measures based on nonlinear dynamics. *IEEE Trans. Audio Speech Lang. Process.*, 17, 1186–1195.

Lopez-de Ipina, K., Alonso, J.-B., Travieso, C. M., Sole-Casals, J., Egiraun, H., Faundez-Zanuy, M., Ezeiza, A., Barroso, N., Ecay-Torres, M., Martinez-Lage, P. et al. (2013). On the selection of non-invasive methods based on speech analysis oriented to automatic Alzheimer disease diagnosis. *Sensors*, 13, 6730–6745.

Jothilakshmi, S. (2014). Automatic system to detect the type of voice pathology. *Appl. Soft Comput.*, 21, 244–249.

Jung, S. Y., Ryu, J.-H., Park, H. S., Chung, S. M., Ryu, D.-R., & Kim, H. S. (2014). Voice change in end-stage renal disease patients after hemodialysis: Correlation of subjective hoarseness and objective acoustic parameters. *J. Voice*, 28, 226–230.

Kaleem, M. F., Ghoraani, B., Guergachi, A., & Krishnan, S. (2011). Telephone quality pathological speech classification using empirical mode decomposition. In *2011 Ann. Int. Conf. IEEE Eng. Med. Biol. Soc.* (pp. 7095–7098).

Karmele López-de-Ipiña, Alonso, J. B., Travieso, C. M., Jordi Solé-Casals, & Lizardui, U. M. D. (2013). On the selection of non-invasive methods based on speech analysis oriented to automatic Alzheimer disease diagnosis. *Sensors*, 5(13), 6730-6745.

Kinnunen, T., & Li, H. (2010). An overview of text-independent speaker recognition: from features to supervectors. *Speech Comm.*, 52(1), 12-40.

King, J. B., Ramig, L. O., Lemke, J. H., & Horii, Y. (1994). Parkinson's disease: longitudinal changes in acoustic parameters of phonation. *J. Med. Speech-Lang. Pathol.*, 2(1), 29-42.

Krawczyk, B. (2016). Learning from imbalanced data: open challenges and future directions. *Prog. Artif. Intell.*, 5, 221–232.

Kumar, R. B., & Bhat, J. S. (2010). Voice in chronic renal failure. *J. Voice*, 24, 690–693.

Le, D., Licata, K., Mercado, E., Persad, C., & Provost, E. M. (2014). Automatic analysis of speech quality for aphasia treatment. In *2014 IEEE Int. Conf. Acoust., Speech Signal Process.* (pp. 4853–4857).

Lee, C. F., Carding, P. N., & Fletcher, M. (2008). The nature and severity of voice disorders in lung cancer patients. *Logop. Phoniatr. Voco.*, 33, 93–103.

Lee, G.-S., Yang, C. C., Wang, C.-P., & Kuo, T. B. (2005). Effect of nasal decongestion on voice spectrum of a nasal consonant-vowel. *J. Voice*, 19, 71–77.

Little, M.A. (2008). Parkinsons data set. Available at http://archive.ics.uci.edu/ml/datasets/Parkinsons.

Little, M. A. (2007). Biomechanically Informed Nonlinear Speech Signal Processing. Ph.D. thesis Dept. Math., Univ. Oxford., Oxford, UK.

Little, M. A., McSharry, P. E., Hunter, E. J., Spielman, J., Ramig, L. O. et al. (2009). Suitability of dysphonia measurements for telemonitoring of Parkinson's disease. *IEEE Trans. Biomed. Eng.*, 56, 1015–1022.

Lopez, V., Fernandez, A., García, S., Palade, V., & Herrera, F. (2013). An insight into classification with imbalanced data: Empirical results and current trends on using data intrinsic characteristics. *Inf. Sci.*, 250, 113–141.

Louren, B.M., Costa, K. M., & da Silva Filho, M. (2014). Voice disorder in cystic fibrosis patients. *PloS one*, 9, e967–69.

Mahbub, U., & Shahnaz, C. (2015). Exploiting wavelet and prosody-related features for the detection of voice disorders. *Am. J. of Biomed. Eng. & Technol.*, 2, 1–13.

Maier, A., Haderlein, T., Stelzle, F., Noth, E., Nkenke, E., Rosanowski, F., Schutzenberger, A., & Schuster, M. (2009). Automatic speech recognition systems for the evaluation of voice and speech disorders in head and neck cancer. *EURASIP J. Audio Speech Music Process.*, 2010, 926–951.

Mandal, I., & Sairam, N. (2013). Accurate telemonitoring of Parkinson's disease diagnosis using robust inference system. *Int. J. Med. Informatics*, 82, 359–377.

Manfredi, C., Lebacq, J., Cantarella, G., Schoentgen, J., Orlandi, S., Bandini, A., & DeJonckere, P. (2017). Smartphones offer new opportunities in clinical voice research. *J. Voice*, 31, 111. e1–111.e7.

Markaki, M., & Stylianou, Y. (2009). Using modulation spectra for voice pathology detection and classification. In *Annu. Int. Conf. IEEE Eng. Med. Biol. Soc.* (pp. 2514–2517).

Markaki, M., & Stylianou, Y. (2011). Voice pathology detection and discrimination based on modulation spectral features. *IEEE Trans. Audio Speech Lang. Process.,* 19, 1938–1948.

Martınez, D., Lleida, E., Ortega, A., Miguel, A., & Villalba, J. (2012). Voice pathology detection on the Saarbrucken Voice Database with calibration and fusion of scores using multifocal toolkit. In Advances in Speech and Language Technologies for Iberian Languages (pp. 99–109). Berlin, Germany: Springer.

Mekyska, J., Janousova, E., Gomez-Vilda, P., Smekal, Z., Rektorova, I., Eliasova, I., Kostalova, M., Mrackova, M., Alonso-Hernandez, J. B., FaundezZanuy, M. et al. (2015). Robust and complex approach of pathological speech signal analysis. *Neurocomputing,* 167, 94–111.

Milken Institute. (2018). The economic burden of chronic disease on the United States. http://www. chronicdiseaseimpact.org/statepdfs/StateFactSheets.pdf (accessed March 2019).

Milone, D. H., Persia, L. E., & Torres, M. E. (2010). Denoising and recognition using hidden Markov models with observation distributions modeled by hidden Markov trees. *Pattern Recogn.,* 43(4), 1577-1589.

Miro, X. A., Bozonnet, S., Evans, N., Fredouille, C., Friedland, G., & Vinyals, O. (2012). Speaker diarization: a review of recent research. *IEEE Trans. Audio Speech Lang. Process.,* 20(2), 356-370.

Moran, R. J., Reilly, R. B., de Chazal, P., & Lacy, P. D. (2006). Telephony based voice pathology assessment using automated speech analysis. *IEEE Trans. Biomed. Eng.,* 53, 468–477.

Muhammad, G., Alsulaiman, M., Ali, Z., Mesallam, T. A., Farahat, M., Malki, K. H., Al-nasheri, A., & Bencherif, M. A. (2017). Voice pathology detection using interlaced derivative pattern on glottal source excitation. *Biomed. Signal Process. Control,* 31, 156–164.

Muhammad, G., Alsulaiman, M., Mahmood, A., & Ali, Z. (2011). Automatic voice disorder classification using vowel formants. In *Proc. IEEE Int. Conf. Multimedia Expo.* (pp. 1–6).

Napierala, K., & Stefanowski, J. (2016). Types of minority class examples and their influence on learning classifiers from imbalanced data. *J. Intell. Inf. Syst.,* 46, 563–597.

Nilashi, M., Ibrahim, O., Ahmadi, H., Shahmoradi, L., & Farahmand, M. (2018). A hybrid intelligent system for the prediction of Parkinson's disease progression using machine learning techniques. *Biocybern. Biomed. Eng.,* 38, 1–15.

Oguz, H., Demirci, M., Safak, M. A., Arslan, N., Islam, A., & Kargin, S. (2007). Effects of unilateral vocal cord paralysis on objective voice measures obtained by Praat. *Eur. Arch. Oto-Rhino-Laryn.,* 264, 257–261.

Orozco-Arroyave, J. R., Belalcazar-Bolanos, E. A., Arias-Londono, J. D., Vargas-Bonilla, J. F., Skodda, S., Rusz, J., Daqrouq, K., Honig, F., & Noth, E. (2015). Characterization methods for the detection of multiple voice disorders: Neurological, functional, and laryngeal diseases. *IEEE J. Biomed. Health Inform.,* 19, 1820–1828.

Orozco-Arroyave, J. R., Murillo-Rendon, S., Alvarez-Meza, A. M., AriasLondono, J. D., Delgado-Trejos, E., Vargas-Bonilla, J., & CastellanosDomınguez, C. G. (2011). Automatic selection of acoustic and non-linear dynamic features in voice signals for hypernasality detection. In *12th Ann. Conf. Int. Speech Commun. Assoc.* (pp. 529–532).

Parsa, V., & Jamieson, D. G. (2000). Identification of pathological voices using glottal noise measures. *J. Speech Lang. Hear Res.,* 43, 469–485.

Poorjam, A. H., Jensen, J. R., Little, M. A., & Christensen, M. G. (2017). Dominant distortion classification for pre-processing of vowels in remote biomedical voice analysis. In *Proc. Interspeech* (pp. 289–293).

Prati, R. C., Batista, G. E., & Silva, D. F. (2015). Class imbalance revisited: a new experimental setup to assess the performance of treatment methods. *Knowl. Inf. Syst.,* 45, 247–270.

Qiu, X., Fu, D., & Fu, Z. (2014). An efficient dimensionality reduction approach for small-sample size and high-dimensional data modeling. *J. Comput.,* 9, 576–580.

Rabiner, L. R. (1989). A tutorial on hidden Markov models and selected applications in speech recognition. *Proc. IEEE,* 77(2), 257-286.

Reilly, R. B., Moran, R. J., & Lacy, P. D. (2004). Voice pathology assessment based on a dialogue system and speech analysis. In *Proc. Am. Assoc. of Artif. Intell. Fall Symp. Dialogue Syst. Health Commun.*

Richardson, F., Reynolds, D., & Dehak, N. (2015). A unified deep neural network for speaker and language recognition. [Online]. Available at https://arxiv.org/abs/1504.00923.

Roy, N., Merrill, R. M., Thibeault, S., Parsa, R. A., Gray, S. D., & Smith, E. M. (2004). Prevalence of voice disorders in teachers and the general population. *J. Speech Lang. Hear Res.*, 47, 281–293.

Rusz, J., Cmejla, R., Ruzickova, H., & Ruzicka, E. (2011). Quantitative acoustic measurements for characterization of speech and voice disorders in early untreated Parkinson's disease. *J. Acoust. Soc. Am.*, 129, 350–367.

Rusz, J., Hlavnicka, J., Tykalova, T., Novotny, M., Dusek, P., Sonka, K., & Ruzicka, E. (2018). Smartphone allows capture of speech abnormalities associated with high risk of developing Parkinson's disease. *IEEE Trans. Neural Syst. Rehabil. Eng.*, 26, 1495–1507.

Saeedi, N. E., & Almasganj, F. (2013). Wavelet adaptation for automatic voice disorders sorting. *Comput. Biol. Med.*, 43, 699–704.

Saeedi, N. E., Almasganj, F., & Torabinejad, F. (2011). Support vector wavelet adaptation for pathological voice assessment. *Comput. Biol. Med.*, 41, 822–828.

Saenz-Lechon, N., Godino-Llorente, J. I., Osma-Ruiz, V., & Gomez-Vilda, P. (2006). Methodological issues in the development of automatic systems for voice pathology detection. *Biomed. Signal Process. Control*, 1, 120–128.

Saudi, A. S. M., Youssif, A. A., & Ghalwash, A. Z. (2012). Computer aided recognition of vocal folds disorders by means of RASTA-PLP. *Comput. Inf. Sci.*, 5, 39–48.

Scalassara, P. R., Maciel, C. D., & Pereira, J. C. (2009). Predictability analysis of voice signals. *IEEE Eng. Med. Biol. Mag.*, 28, 30–34.

Schulz, G. M., & Grant, M. K. (2000). Effects of speech therapy and pharmacologic and surgical treatments on voice and speech in Parkinson's disease: a review of the literature. *J. Commun. Disord.*, 33, 59–88.

Shastry, A., Balasubramanium, R. K., & Acharya, P. R. (2014). Voice analysis in individuals with chronic obstructive pulmonary disease. *Int. J. Phonosurg. Laryngol.*, 4, 45–49.

Shrivastav, R., Rosenbek, J. C., Harnsberger, J. D., & Anand, S. (2014). Systems and methods of screening for medical states using speech and other vocal behaviors.

Song, E., Ryu, J., & Kang, H. G. (2013). Speech enhancement for pathological voice using time-frequency trajectory excitation modeling. *Signal & Inform. Proc. Assoc. Summit & Conf.*

Teager, H., & Teager, S. (1990). Evidence for nonlinear sound production mechanisms in the vocal tract. *Speech Prod. Speech Model.*, 55, 241–261.

The US Burden of Disease Collaborators (2018). The state of us health, 1990-2016: Burden of diseases, injuries, and risk factors among us states. *JAMA*, 319, 1444–1472.

Ting, K. M. (2000). A comparative study of cost-sensitive boosting algorithms. In *Proc. Int. Conf. Mach. Learn.* (pp. 983–990).

Titze, I. R. (1994). Principles of Voice Production. Englewood Cliffs, NJ, USA: Prentice Hall.

Tsanas, A. (2012) Accurate telemonitoring of Parkinson's disease symptom severity using nonlinear speech signal processing and statistical machine learning. Ph.D. thesis Dept. Appl. Math., Univ. Oxford., Oxford, UK.

Tsanas, A., & Little, M. A. (2009). Parkinsons telemonitoring data set. Available at http://archive.ics.uci.edu/ml/datasets/Parkinsons+ Telemonitoring.

Tsanas, A., & Little, M. A. (2012). Parkinson's voice initiative. Available at http://www.parkinsonsvoice.org/vision.php.

Tsanas, A., Little, M. A., McSharry, P. E., & Ramig, L. O. (2010). Accurate telemonitoring of Parkinson's disease progression by noninvasive speech tests. *IEEE Trans. Biomed. Eng.*, 57, 884–893.

Tsanas, A., Little, M. A., McSharry, P. E., & Ramig, L. O. (2011). Nonlinear speech analysis algorithms mapped to a standard metric achieve clinically useful quantification of average Parkinson's disease symptom severity. *J. R. Soc. Interface,* 8, 842–855.

Tsanas, A., Little, M. A., McSharry, P. E., Spielman, J., & Ramig, L. O. (2012). Novel speech signal processing algorithms for high-accuracy classification of Parkinson's disease. *IEEE Trans. Biomed. Eng.,* 59, 1264–1271.

Vaizman, Y., McFee, B., & Lanckriet, G. (2014). Codebook-based audio feature representation for music information retrieval. *IEEE/ACM Trans. Audio Speech Lang. Process.,* 22, 1483–1493.

Vasquez, J., Orozco, J. R., & Noeth, E. (2017). Convolutional neural network to model articulation impairments in patients with Parkinson's disease. In *Proc. Interspeech* (pp. 314–318).

Vikram, C., & Umarani, K. (2013). Pathological voice analysis to detect neurological disorders using MFCC and SVM. *Int. J. Adv. Electr. Electron. Eng.,* 2, 87–91.

Wang, J. Q., Gao, X., Wang, J., Chen, F., Yang, Y., & Hu, H. Y. (2004). The Application of Voice Acoustic Analysis in Evaluation of Electronic Laryngoscope Operation. *Suzhou Univ. J. Med. Sci.,* 24(6), 878-880.

Wang, Z., Yu, P., Yan, N., Wang, L., & Ng, M. L. (2016). Automatic assessment of pathological voice quality using multidimensional acoustic analysis based on the GRBAS scale. *J. Signal Process. Sys.,* 82, 241–251.

Wasikowski, M., & Chen, X.-w (2010). Combating the small sample class imbalance problem using feature selection. *IEEE Trans. Knowl. Data Eng.,* 22, 1388–1400.

Whitehill, T. L., Ciocca, V., Chan, J. C.-T., & Samman, N. (2006). Acoustic analysis of vowels following glossectomy. *Clin. Linguist. Phon.,* 20, 135–140.

Williams, D. F. (2014). Communication sciences and disorders: an introduction to the professions. London, United Kingdom: Psychology Press.

Xu, Y., Yang, Z., Zhang, Y., Pan, X., & Wang, L. (2016). A maximum margin and minimum volume hyper-spheres machine with pinball loss for imbalanced data classification. *Knowl. Based Syst.,* 95, 75–85.

Yata, K., & Aoshima, M. (2012). Effective PCA for high-dimension, low-sample size data with noise reduction via geometric representations. *J. Multivariate Anal.,* 105, 193–215.

Zhang, H., Wang, A., Li, D., & Xu, W. (2018). DeepVoice: A voiceprint-based mobile health framework for Parkinson's disease identification. In *2018 IEEE EMBS Int. Conf. on Biomed. Health Inform.* (pp. 214–217).

Zhang, L., & Lin, X. (2013). Some considerations of classification for high dimension low-sample size data. *Stat. Methods Med. Res.,* 22, 537–550.

Zhang, X., Tao, Z., Zhao, H., & Xu, T. (2017). Pathological voice recognition by deep neural network. In *2017 4th Int. Con. Syst. Inform.* (pp. 464–468).

Zhou, X., Garcia-Romero, D., Mesgarani, N., Stone, M., Espy-Wilson, C., & Shamma, S. (2012). Automatic intelligibility assessment of pathologic speech in head and neck cancer based on auditory-inspired spectro-temporal modulations. In *Proc. Interspeech* (pp. 542–545)

Chapter 2
Pathological Voice Acquisition

Abstract In pathological voice analysis, voice acquisition is of great importance since the quality of the voice has great impacts on the performance of voice analysis. In particular, the influence of SNR (signal-to-noise ratio) and sampling rate during recording are two key factors that require investigation.

Firstly, according to previous literature (Das, Expert Syst. Appl. 37, 1568–1572, 2010), a pathological voice often displays signs in the high frequency band, coinciding with the frequency range where numerous types of noise may lie. When voices are recorded with large amount of noise around, indicating a low environmental SNR, the pathological characteristics may be mixed with noise and the pathological voice analysis under this circumstance will be adversely affected. It should be noted that particular attention on the environmental SNR is meaningful since the real acoustic environment for pathological voice analysis is more diverse and complex. Thus, the influence of environmental SNR should be deeply researched further. Second, when pathological voice often shows signs in the high frequency band, the selection of sampling rate will be critical in order to capture the discriminative information for the screening of pathological voice. Besides, sampling rate may be an essential aspect that determines the cost of sampling device. In the next part, we focus on the second one and try to reveal the optimal selection of sampling rate based on six metrics, especially for Parkinson's disease.

Keywords Parkinson's disease · Sampling rate · Voice acquisition · Voice analysis

In pathological voice analysis, voice acquisition is of great importance since the quality of the voice has great impacts on the performance of voice analysis. In particular, the influence of SNR (signal-to-noise ratio) and sampling rate during recording are two key factors that require investigation.

Firstly, according to previous literature (Das 2010), a pathological voice often displays signs in the high frequency band, coinciding with the frequency range where numerous types of noise may lie. When voices are recorded with large amount of noise around, indicating a low environmental SNR, the pathological characteristics may be mixed with noise and the pathological voice analysis under this

© Springer Nature Singapore Pte Ltd. 2020
D. Zhang, K. Wu, *Pathological Voice Analysis*,
https://doi.org/10.1007/978-981-32-9196-6_2

circumstance will be adversely affected. It should be noted that particular attention on the environmental SNR is meaningful since the real acoustic environment for pathological voice analysis is more diverse and complex. Thus, the influence of environmental SNR should be deeply researched further. Secondly, when pathological voice often shows signs in the high frequency band, the selection of sampling rate will be critical in order to capture the discriminative information for the screening of pathological voice. Besides, sampling rate may be an essential aspect that determines the cost of sampling device.

In this chapter, we focus on the second one and try to reveal the optimal selection of sampling rate based on six metrics, especially for Parkinson's disease.

2.1 Introduction

Parkinson's disease (PD) is a neurological disorder that profoundly affects the daily life of patients and their families. Due to its high morbidity, PD has received increasing attention worldwide. It was estimated by Parkinson's Disease Foundation that around 7–10 million people worldwide are affected by PD. Traditional methods to diagnose and monitor PD have some major disadvantages. First, patients have to go to hospital frequently, which is inconvenient and even impossible for patients with PD (PWP) since their disability often increases with the aggravation of PD. Second, diagnostic results by doctors are subjective. In fact, diagnosis depends heavily on the doctors' experience and thus different doctors may give diverse diagnostic results for the same patient (Zhan et al. 2016). Finally, current diagnosis needs the assistance of some advanced imaging tools like SPECT scans (Brooks 2007; Ho et al. 1999), which are not always affordable for both patients and hospitals, especially in rural areas. These weaknesses motivate researchers to investigate alternative ways to diagnose and monitor PD so that current shortcomings can be avoided or alleviated (Little 2007; Tsanas 2012; Little et al. 2009).

Recent studies show that PD patients display a certain extent of vocal impairment (Ho et al. 1999). Researchers in the artificial intelligence field, therefore, attempt to explore the potential to analyze voice recording for PD assessment (Little 2007; Tsanas 2012; Little et al. 2009; Tsanas et al. 2010, 2012; Sakar et al. 2013; Bocklet et al. 2011). For simplicity, PD assessment (monitoring) through voice analysis is termed as PDVA thereafter. In Tsanas et al. (2012), the accuracy to discriminate PWPs from healthy controls by automatically analyzing the collected sustained vowels reached almost 99%. Moreover, it was demonstrated that voice analysis can also be employed to predict and track the ongoing PD symptom severity (Little et al. 2009). These promising outcomes make it possible to perform remote diagnosis and monitoring of PD, in which scenario PWPs can be diagnosed and monitored objectively at home (Tsanas 2012). Besides, it is essential to point out that PDVA is non-invasive and the financial cost of voice recording device is relatively low. Consequently, the three weaknesses of traditional PD diagnosis can be handled by this modern way.

Despite the encouraging results, there is a long way to go before putting PDVA into clinical use due to the limitations existing in current studies. In the first place, the reported classification accuracy is based on experimental results implemented on rather small databases. In Tsanas et al. (2012), the employed database consists of 10 healthy controls and 33 PWPs only. The limited sample size casts uncertainty for the PDVA performance in practical use. Hence, it is essential to explore the PDVA performance in terms of accuracy and robustness on a larger database. Secondly, the influence of environmental SNR (signal-to-noise ratio) during recording is yet for investigation. According to previous literature (Das 2010), a pathological voice often displays signs in the high frequency band, coinciding with the frequency range where numerous types of noise may lie. When voices are recorded with large amount of noise around, indicating a low environmental SNR, the pathological characteristics may be mixed with noise and the PDVA under this circumstance will be adversely affected. It should be noted that particular attention on the environmental SNR is meaningful since the real acoustic environment for PDVA is more diverse and complex. Thus, the influence of environmental SNR should be deeply researched further. Thirdly, there is no verified guideline on the voice collection. When collecting voice, some key components must be determined, such as the sampling rate and quantization bit. However, rare investigation has been carried out to explore the impacts of these factors. To speed up the development of PDVA, the preceding limitations must be carefully considered. In this paper, we focus on the third weakness and try to reveal the optimal selection of sampling rate for PDVA.

When voice is captured with a microphone, it should then be digitalized, in which the sampling rate (SR) is one crucial parameter. However, SR varies largely in the literature of PDVA. For example, the SR in Sakar et al. (2013) was as high as 96 kHz, while it was set as 48 kHz in Bocklet et al. (2011) and Rusz et al. (2011) and 24 kHz in Tsanas et al. (2011). In the following works (Rahn et al. 2007; Shao et al. 2010; Bolat and Bolat Sert 2010), the SR was fixed as 20 kHz. Besides, in the majority of published studies (Tsanas 2012; Tsanas et al. 2012, 2014a; Midi et al. 2008; Orozco-Arroyave et al. 2014; Kent et al. 2003; Benba et al. 2014; Dubey et al. 2015; Karimi Rouzbahani and Daliri 2011; Das 2010), voice was sampled at 44.1 kHz. Given the large variability of the chosen sampling rates in this field, it would be beneficial to carefully consider their effect and possible limitations. Even though a concerned statement in Tsanas et al. (2012) recommended that the SR should be in the range of 20–100 kHz, there are no experimental or theoretical evidences provided to support this declaration. Therefore, we are motivated to perform a deeper exploration into the impacts of sampling rate. We remark that although PD assessment is used as a paradigm here, this investigation might be used to guide related biomedical applications where speech signals are used.

The influence of SR has been considered in several applications, including ECG delineation (Simon et al. 2007), speech recognition (Ssnderson and Paliwal 1997), and two other automatic systems (Li et al. 2010; Ma et al. 2015). Previous works can be divided into three categories. First, some works are dealing with the sampling rate inconsistencies, which were termed as sampling rate compensations. The inconsistency occurs when the sampling frequency in training stage of an automatic system is different from that in the testing stage. Second, how sampling rate affects the performance of many tasks is studied. Third, since low sampling rate often results in low-quality signals, researchers have also sought super-resolution techniques to reconstruct signal of high sampling rate. Evidently, sampling rate plays an important role for many automatic systems. Moreover, it should be reminded that the famous Nyquist theory alone is not enough to determine the optimal sampling rate. Although the theory provides the relation between the lowest sampling rate needed and the cut-off frequency in a signal, the criterion to decide the cut-off frequency is application-oriented. For instance, in the case of telephone communication, the cut-off frequency is assigned as 3.4 kHz and a sampling rate of 8 kHz will be enough. However, the suggested sampling frequency in speech recognition is much higher than 8 kHz (Ssnderson and Paliwal 1997). Hence, an in-depth exploration of the digitalization parameter optimization is necessary.

To explore the influence of SR, we consider measures in different levels. First of all, the accuracy of PDVA, which refers to the classification rate of discriminating PWP from the healthy control, is the main criteria. Secondly, measure in feature level is adopted since the quality of the extracted features depends on the quality of the recorded voice, of which SR is one of the key aspects. Hence, correlations among features for voice of different SR are investigated. Thirdly, measures in signal level, such as information entropy and reconstruction error, are included. Finally, we also consider hardware-level metrics like storage and computational cost since they may impose limits to the wider extension of PDVA, especially on smartphone platform. These four levels are considered to achieve a comprehensive investigation.

In this section, we first established a database consisting of voice from both healthy controls and the PWPs. Then experiments were designed to investigate the influence of SR for PDVA by using six metrics from four levels: information quantity, reconstruction error, classification accuracy, feature correlations, storage burden, and the computational cost. With the empirical conclusions, we hope that it may provide a basic guideline for the selection of SR for PDVA.

More details about this section, such as metrics adopted and experimental results, are well demonstrated in literature (Wu et al. 2018).

2.2 Database Description

To evaluate the influence of SR on PDVA, a database consisting of voice samples from both PWPs and healthy controls is built. Here all samples are collected using the same recording device and the block diagram of our data acquisition system is shown in Fig. 2.1, where the hardware equipment includes soundproof room, microphone, sound card, and computer. Figure 2.2 presents more details about the system. Since the voice recording can be easily contaminated by noise, which may affect the performance of pathological voice analysis, all voice is recorded in a soundproofed room with a size of 1.25 m × 1.015 m × 2.10 m. As to the microphone adopted, AKG C214 is selected with the reasons listed as follows: First, C214 is a

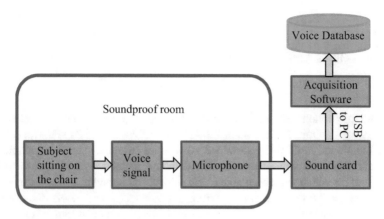

Fig. 2.1 The diagram of voice signal acquisition

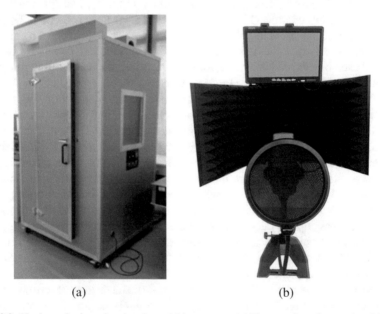

(a)   (b)

Fig. 2.2 Hardware in the voice signal acquisition system. (**a**) The soundproof room, in which the subjects are asked to sit on a chair and sustain vowels. (**b**) From top to bottom are screen (show guidelines for subjects), soundproof mask, and microphone

cardioid condenser microphone so that the sounds from other directions can be attenuated. Second, the frequency response of C214 is relatively smooth and flat. Third, low self-noise and therefore high SNR (signal-to-noise ratio) are also key features. Finally, the high sensitivity of C214 has enabled the suitability. More information about AKG C214 can be referred in AKG Acoustics GmbH (2015). When recording, the subjects were asked to sit comfortably on a chair with adjustable height, with a distance of 20 cm (as suggested in the manual of AKG C214)

Table 2.1 Comparison of clinical variables between healthy individuals (controls) and patients with PD (cases)

Item	Healthy	PD
Number	102	34 (all on medication)
Male/female	52/50	24/10
Age	19–64	40–84

from the microphone ahead. The sound card used in the system is Roland UA-55, and the sampling rate and the quantization bit are 192 kHz and 24 bits, respectively.

As mentioned in Chap. 1, sustained vowels are commonly used in pathological voice analysis. The vowels used in this database include /a:/, /ə/, and /i:/ with a duration of 2 s which was acceptable for all subjects including patients. If a recording does not meet the requirements (a wrong pronunciation or a short duration), the subject was asked to re-sustain the vowels until a qualified recording is collected. In all, we have built a voice database collected from Guangdong Provincial Hospital of Traditional Chinese Medicine (Guangzhou, China). In total, the sample numbers of PWPs and healthy controls (HC) are 34 and 102, respectively. Some information about the subjects is listed in Table 2.1. The health labels were decided by physical examinations, whereas the PD patients were diagnosed and confirmed by two doctors based on clinical history, neurological examination, and imaging (magnetic resonance imaging (MRI) and SPECT). As noted, the sampling rate used in the sampling is as high as 192 kHz and we explain the reason in the following.

To analyze the influence of SR on PDVA, voices of various sampling rates should be included. There are two methods to obtain data of this requirement. The first is to ask each subject to pronounce the vowel several times, with each time using a different SR. However, it not only consumes more time in voice recording, but also brings difficulty in finding the influences of SR since his/her way to pronounce a word cannot be exactly the same when recorded with different sampling rates. Another way is to ask each subject to sustain the voice only once and then synthesize voices of other sampling rates using the recorded voice. In this way, sampling rate will be the only factor that leads to the difference among voices of different sampling rates. In addition, it is more efficient for participants. Due to the advantages, this second recording approach is applied.

Downsampling and upsampling are two possible methods to synthesize voice of a different sampling rate. When voice of high SR cannot be accurately constructed by upsampling a voice of low SR, downsampling a voice of high SR can generate the corresponding voice of low SR precisely. Hence, we choose to record voice with a high SR and then construct voice of other SR by downsampling. For our aim, the sampling rate used in recording is set as 192 kHz (using the professional sound card Roland UA-55), and then voice samples of lower sampling rates (in previous works, the rate varies from 20 to 96 kHz) can be generated.

To generate voices of lower sampling rates, the recorded voices are downsampled using the algorithm proposed in Crochiere and Rabiner (1983). Note that a low pass FIR (finite impulse response) filter smoothed by the Kaiser window is employed before downsampling to avoid anti-aliasing. The sampling rates in our comparison are listed as follows in a descending order:

$$R = \{192, 96, 48, 44.1, 32, 25, 24, 20, 16, 8, 4, 2, 1\}\text{kHz.} \tag{2.1}$$

In this set, the first 10 frequencies are commonly used in digitalization. The last three sampling rates are included to show the tendency of influence.

2.3   Experimental Results

2.3.1   Metric 1: Information Entropy (Signal Level)

Information entropy is a measure used in the theory of communication to indicate the quantity of information (Stone 2014). For a continuous random variable Y, the differential entropy is often applied:

$$H(Y) = -\int_{-\infty}^{+\infty} p(y) \ln p(y) dy, \tag{2.2}$$

where $p(y)$ is the continuous probability density. With the entropy measure defined in Eq. (2.2), we first calculated the entropy for all subjects of all sampling rates in set R. Then the average entropy of voices of the same SR is computed. Due to the loss of high frequency detailed information in downsampling, the entropy of a downsampled voice should decrease, comparing with the raw signal originally recorded using a sampling rate of 192 kHz. Figure 2.3 shows that with the increase of sampling rate, entropy grows rapidly at first and then remains almost the same when the sampling rate is larger than 16 kHz. Besides, the chosen sampling rate

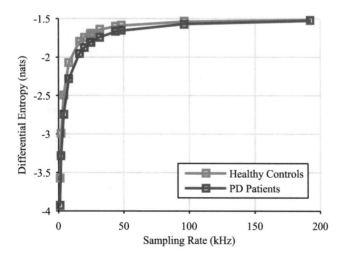

Fig. 2.3 (color online) Comparison of differential entropy between healthy individuals (controls) and patients with PD (cases) at different sampling rates

should be no less than 16 kHz to avoid information loss. Besides, little information gain can be obtained when the sampling rate exceeds 16 kHz.

2.3.2   Metric 2: Reconstruction Error (Signal Level)

In this section, we employ the mean absolute reconstruction error (MAE), which is another metric in signal level based on waveform directly, to measure the detail loss.

With a voice of a lower sampling rate, for instance, 16 kHz, the corresponding voice of 192 kHz can be reconstructed, even with certain amounts of errors. The process of reconstruction is actually upsampling involving zero interpolation and low pass filtering (Crochiere and Rabiner 1983). The low pass filter used remains the same as in Sect. 2.2. All generated voices of lower rates are upsampled to 192 kHz, which is the actual sampling rate in recording. Suppose that s_o is the recorded voice and s_{re} is the reconstructed one, then MAE for this reconstruction is computed as follows, where L denotes the length of s_o.

$$E = \frac{1}{L} \sum_{i=1}^{L} | s_o - s_{re} | . \tag{2.3}$$

Likewise, MAEs for samples at each SR are averaged. The influence of sampling rate on reconstruction error is displayed in Fig. 2.4. It can be seen that MAE increases when the sampling rate gap is larger. For SR varying from 16 to 192 kHz, the reconstruction error is almost negligible for healthy controls and PD patients (all voices have been normalized into the range $[-1, 1]$). By contrast, when

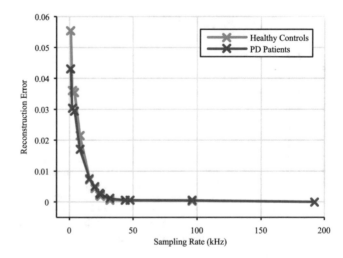

Fig. 2.4 (color online) Comparison of reconstruction errors between healthy individuals (controls) and patients with PD (cases) at different sampling rates

SR drops to less than 16 kHz, the reconstruction error grows dramatically with the decrease of sampling rate. As a conclusion, the sampling rate should be no lower than 16 kHz.

2.3.3   Metric 3: Feature Correlation (Feature Level)

In this section, we perform analysis in feature level to guide the sampling rate selection. Since voices of PWPs are often hoarse, breathy, and less articulated, several types of acoustic features were proposed to detect PD (Tsanas 2012; Little et al. 2009; Tsanas et al. 2012; Bocklet et al. 2011; Rusz et al. 2011). In Godino-Llorente et al. (2006), the authors proposed to adopt the short-term Mel frequency cepstral coefficients (MFCC) for PD assessment. Similarly, MFCC features have been employed (Tsanas 2012; Fraile et al. 2009; Jafari 2013; Kapoor and Sharma 2011) for disease (including PD) differentiation purposes. Meanwhile, other MFCC related features are added, including the 0-th MFCC coefficient, log-energy, as well as the first and second derivatives of MFCC. Each recording is represented with the mean and standard derivations of MFCC related features across all frames.

First, the abovementioned features are extracted for each recording, including both the recorded and generated ones. Eventually, the mean correlation matrix for HC (PD) group is gained by averaging over all healthy subjects (PD patients). Let v_{si} denote the normalized feature vector extracted from voice of the sth subject and ith sampling rate (in set R). For clarity, the way to derive the mean correlation matrix is formulated below.

$$\rho_{ij} = \frac{1}{S} \sum_{s=1}^{S} v_{si}{}^{\mathrm{T}} v_{sj}. \tag{2.4}$$

Here the sample number S equals to 102 (34) for HC (PD) group and ρ_{ij} represents the averaged correlation between the feature sets of ith and jth sampling rate. In Figs. 2.5 and 2.6, the average correlation matrix for HC and PD groups is shown as images, respectively, with the color denoting the correlation value. The pairwise correlation is highly controlled by the sampling rate gap: the larger the gap is, the lower the correlation is. Another pivotal finding is that the pairwise correlation is relatively high when both sampling rates are in the range of 16–192 kHz. Specifically, the average pairwise correlation coefficient in this range is 0.960 for HC group. However, when the SR range extends by adding the next sampling rate in set R, which is 8 kHz, it turns out that the mean correlation value in this range for healthy subjects drops dramatically to 0.886. The feature correlation for PD group shows a similar result. To this end, there are strong correlations among features of different sampling rates ranging from 16 to 192 kHz, while the correlation decreases greatly when the sampling rate 8 kHz is added. Hence, we should choose a sampling rate that is no less than 16 kHz.

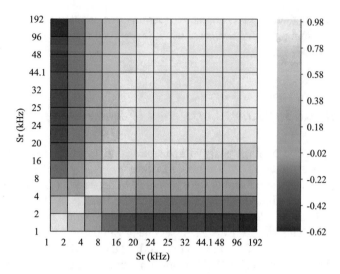

Fig. 2.5 (color online) Pairwise correlation among features of different sampling rates for healthy controls

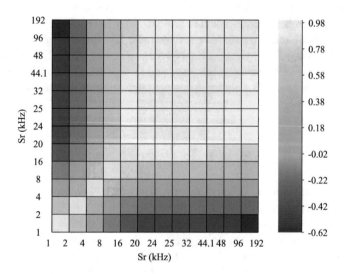

Fig. 2.6 (color online) Pairwise correlation among features of different sampling rates for PD group

2.3.4 Metric 4: Classification Accuracy (System Level)

In this part, we investigate the effect of sampling rate on classification accuracy of PDVA. The same procedure is performed for each sampling rate. First, MFCC related features are extracted following the description in Sect. 2.3.3. Second, feature

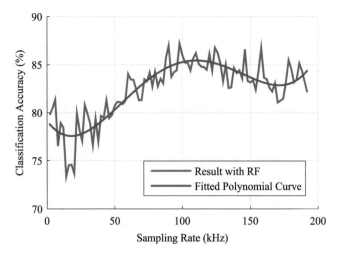

Fig. 2.7 (color online) The impact of sampling rate on classification accuracy

dataset is split into training and testing sets with a three-fold cross validation in the classification stage. Besides, we apply the ADASYN technique (He et al. 2008) to generate synthetic PD samples to make the sample sizes for PD and healthy control class balanced. Third, Random Forest (RF, Fernandez-Delgado et al. 2014) is used to discriminate PWPs from the healthy subjects (parameters in RF keep the same for all sampling rates).

To get a better insight into the influence of sampling rate on the performance of PDVA, the SR of our experiments varies from 2 to 192 kHz with a step size of 2 kHz. The effect of SR on classification accuracy is illustrated in Fig. 2.7, including the best fitted polynomial curve (in a least square sense) to find out the overall tendency. The accuracy rate drops when the SR increases from 2 to 20 kHz. Then, the rate increases with the sampling rate until the SR exceeds 106 kHz. Especially, the sharp decrease in the range of 14–16 kHz might be caused by decrease of the relative difference between the spectrum of two classes (PD and HC). Finally, the accuracy rate decreases gradually. Still, the accuracy is over 85% when the SR is in the range of 94–118 kHz. Considering the current market of sound card, a sampling rate of 96 kHz may be proper. Additionally, it should be noted that the influence of sampling rate may change when different features and vowels are applied.

2.3.5 Metric 5: Computational Cost (Hardware Level)

Large computational complexity will limit the extension of PDVA. Hence, the optimization of sampling rate needs to consider the computational cost. In this part, we compare the running time of PDVA for recordings of different sampling rates. The two main steps in PDVA are feature extraction and prediction

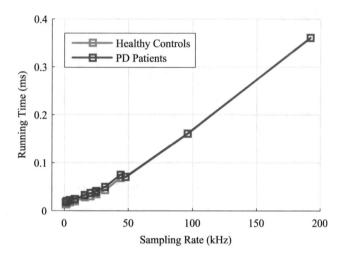

Fig. 2.8 (color online) Comparison of running time between healthy individuals (controls) and patients with PD (cases) at different sampling rates

(classification or regression). The features used here are MFCC and its extensions as described in Sect. 2.3.3, and they keep the same dimension. Since MFCC features are calculated on frame bases with a frame length of 30 ms, a higher SR indicates more data points. Hence, a higher sampling rate results in higher computational cost.

Given a recording, the elapsed time to extract features is measured and then normalized by the number of frames. Then the mean normalized running time for each sampling rate is computed by averaging over all healthy (PD) samples of the same sampling rate. The experiment is carried out in same hardware. The average computational costs under different sampling rates for two groups are presented in Fig. 2.8. As with our analysis, the running time drops with the decrease of sampling rate, indicating the benefit of a lower SR.

2.3.6   Metric 6: Storage Cost (Hardware Level)

A high SR needs more space to store the recordings, which may be particularly challenging when PDVA is applied on the smartphone platform. Moreover, storage size shall be considered when telemedicine technology is applied for PDVA. Hence, the storage cost is also considered as a metric to assess the influence of different SR.

When the recording duration is fixed, the demanding storage size is linearly proportional to SR. Here the quantization bit is assigned to 24 bit and the length for each recording is 2 s. Then in theory, each recording sampled with a frequency S_r can be calculated as follows, where the unit for storage C is byte:

$$C = 6S_r. \tag{2.5}$$

According to Eq. (2.5), the bytes allocated for each recording is 1124 Kbyte with the initial sampling rate of 192 kHz; meanwhile, the cost drops to 93.75 Kb when the recording is downsampled at 16 kHz. Clearly, a lower SR is more beneficial if the storage cost is considered.

2.3.7   Discussion and Guideline on the Sampling Rate Selection

Based on the former six experiments, a basic guideline for the sampling rate selection is summarized in Table 2.2. It is observed that the results with the first three metrics indicate that a sampling rate of 16 kHz is enough. However, the analysis in Sect. 2.3.4 demonstrates that this value of SR shows a low accuracy rate.

In fact, while downsampling with a lower sampling rate, such as 16 kHz, can maintain most information in the signal, detail in the high frequency band are lost. Unfortunately, the energy in high frequency band is generally increased in pathological voice, caused by incomplete vocal fold closure (Tsanas 2012). Hence, both the approximate (in the low frequency band) and the detailed information (in the high frequency band) in voice should be kept to discriminate PWPs from HC more accurately.

Based on the former analysis, one can choose a proper sampling rate accordingly for different applications. For instance, when conducting PDVA in a smartphone platform, a lower sampling rate should be chosen because of limitations in computational and storage. Otherwise, a sampling rate of 96 kHz should be used to obtain the highest detection rate.

It must be emphasized that there exist some limitations about this guideline and one should be cautious to apply the conclusion directly. First of all, if a different vowel or continuous speech is used in experiments, the sampling rate may affect PDVA differently. Secondly, when another disease is concerned, the guideline in Table 2.2 is no longer applicable, similar conclusion was also mentioned in paper (Kasuya et al. 1986). Thirdly, more metrics measuring the influence of SR may be added according to the specialized application demands. For instance, one may add a metric concerning the accuracy and reliability of F0 estimation to study the influence

Metric names	Suggested sampling rate
Information entropy	$\geq$16 kHz
Reconstruction error	$\geq$16 kHz
Feature correlation	$\geq$16 kHz
Classification rate	In the range of 94–118 kHz
Computational cost	As low as possible
Storage cost	As low as possible

Table 2.2 Metrics and the suggested sampling rates

of SR in the assessment of voice pathology, as in the works (Deliyski et al. 2005; Tsanas et al. 2014b). Despite these limitations, we claimed that our work still provides a basic framework and different levels of metrics for the study of the influence of sampling rate. In particular, given a specific setting, we may investigate the impact of sampling rate using the same metrics proposed in this chapter.

2.4 Summary

In this chapter, the influence of sampling rate on PDVA is studied to form a basic guideline on the selection of sampling rate. For this purpose, a database for PDVA is collected including voices from both healthy controls and PD patients, for which special considerations have been taken to enable the optimization of sampling rate. Then experiments to measure the impacts of sampling rate are implemented. In addition, the guideline to set sampling rate for PDVA is presented, which may help to determine the sampling rate according to the demands of different applications. In the future, we aim to further conduct researches on issues that hinder the process of putting PDVA into practical use. For instance, the influence of environmental SNR in particular will be studied.

Parkinson's diagnosis through voice analysis (PDVA) has been attracting increasing attention. In this section, the influence of sampling rate on PDVA is studied. By analyzing the main difficulties that hamper the development of PDVA, the significance of seeking guidelines on sampling rate is discussed. Then voices from both healthy controls and patients with Parkinson's disease are recorded, for which the sampling rate used is given special consideration. Recordings of other sampling rates are generated via downsampling the recorded voices. Then it is proposed to adopt six metrics from four levels to assess the impacts of sampling rate, which are information entropy, reconstruction error, feature correlation, classification accuracy, computational cost, and storage cost. Through extensive experiments, basic guideline to seek an appropriate sampling rate is provided. It is concluded that a sampling rate of 96 kHz is preferred when no limits of storage and computational costs are imposed. However, a lower sampling rate may be needed if the storage size and computational complexity are the main concerns.

References

AKG Acoustics GmbH (2015). *C214 professional large-diaphragm condenser microphone.* https:// www.akg.com/on/demandware.static/-/Sites-masterCatalog_Harman/default/dwa4360d70/ pdfs/AKG_C214_Manual.pdf.

Benba, A., Jilbab, A., & Hammouch, A. (2014). Voice analysis for detecting persons with Parkinson's disease using PLP and VQ. *J. Theor. Appl. Inf. Technol., 70.*

Bocklet, T., Noth, E., Stemmer, G., Ruzickova, H., & Rusz, J. (2011). Detection of persons with Parkinson's disease by acoustic, vocal, and prosodic analysis. In *Automatic Speech Recognition and Understanding (ASRU), 2011 IEEE Workshop on* (pp. 478–483). IEEE.

Bolat, B., & Bolat Sert, S. (2010). Classification of Parkinson's disease by using voice measurements. *Int. J. Reasoning-based Intell. Syst.*, *2*, 279–284.

Brooks, D. J. (2007). Assessment of Parkinson's disease with imaging. *Parkinsonism Relat. Disord.*, *13*, S268–S275.

Crochiere, R. E., & Rabiner, L. R. (1983). *Multirate digital signal processing* volume 18. Prentice-hall Englewood Cliffs, NJ.

Das, R. (2010). A comparison of multiple classification methods for diagnosis of Parkinson disease. *Expert Syst. Appl.*, *37*, 1568–1572.

Deliyski, D. D., Shaw, H. S., & Evans, M. K. (2005). Influence of sampling rate on accuracy and reliability of acoustic voice analysis. *Logop. Phoniatr. Voco.*, *30*, 55–62.

Dubey, H., Goldberg, J. C., Abtahi, M., Mahler, L., & Mankodiya, K. (2015). EchoWear: smartwatch technology for voice and speech treatments of patients with Parkinson's disease. In *Proceedings of the conference on Wireless Health* (p. 15). ACM.

Fernandez-Delgado, M., Cernadas, E., Barro, S., & Amorim, D. (2014). Do we need hundreds of classifiers to solve real world classification problems. *J. Mach. Learn. Res.*, *15*, 3133–3181.

Fraile, R., Saenz-Lechon, N., Godino-Llorente, J. I., Osma-Ruiz, V., & Fredouille, C. (2009). Mfcc-based remote pathology detection on speech transmitted through the telephone channel - impact of linear distortions: Band limitation, frequency response and noise. In *Proceedings of the International Conference on Bio-Inspired Systems and Signal Processing* (pp. 41–48).

Godino-Llorente, J. I., Gomez-Vilda, P., & Blanco-Velasco, M. (2006). Dimensionality reduction of a pathological voice quality assessment system based on Gaussian mixture models and short-term cepstral parameters. *IEEE Trans. Biomed. Eng.*, *53*, 1943–1953.

He, H., Bai, Y., Garcia, E. A., & Li, S. (2008). ADASYN: Adaptive synthetic sampling approach for imbalanced learning. In *Neural Networks, 2008. IJCNN 2008. (IEEE World Congress on Computational Intelligence). IEEE International Joint Conference on* (pp. 1322–1328). IEEE.

Ho, A. K., Iansek, R., Marigliani, C., Bradshaw, J. L., & Gates, S. (1999). Speech impairment in a large sample of patients with Parkinson's disease. *Behav. Neurol.*, *11*, 131–137.

Jafari, A. (2013). Classification of Parkinson's disease patients using nonlinear phonetic features and mel-frequency cepstral analysis. *Biomed. Eng.: Appl., Basis Commun.*, *25*, 1350001.

Kapoor, T., & Sharma, R. (2011). Parkinson's disease diagnosis using mel-frequency cepstral coefficients and vector quantization. *Int. J. Comput. Appl.*, *14*, 43–46.

Karimi Rouzbahani, H., & Daliri, M. R. (2011). Diagnosis of Parkinson's disease in human using voice signals. *Basic Clin. Neurosci.*, *2*, 12–20.

Kasuya, H., Ogawa, S., Mashima, K., & Ebihara, S. (1986). Normalized noise energy as an acoustic measure to evaluate pathologic voice. *J. Acoust. Soc. Am.*, *80*, 1329–1334.

Kent, R., Vorperian, H., Kent, J., & Duffy, J. R. (2003). Voice dysfunction in dysarthria: application of the multi-dimensional voice program. *J. Commun. Disord.*, *36*, 281–306.

Li, G., Li, Y., Zhang, Z., Geng, Y., & Zhou, R. (2010). Selection of sampling rate for EMG pattern recognition based prosthesis control. In *Engineering in Medicine and Biology Society (EMBC), 2010 Annual International Conference of the IEEE* (pp. 5058–5061). IEEE.

Little, M. (2007). Biomechanically informed, nonlinear speech signal processing. university of oxford.

Little, M. A., McSharry, P. E., Hunter, E. J., Spielman, J., Ramig, L. O. et al. (2009). Suitability of dysphonia measurements for telemonitoring of Parkinson's disease. *IEEE Trans. Biomed. Eng.*, *56*, 1015–1022.

Ma, Z. B., Yang, Y., Zhou, F., & Jian-Hua, X. (2015). A real-time fatigue driving detection system design and implementation. In *Advanced Communication Technology (ICACT), 2015 17th International Conference on* (pp. 483–488). IEEE.

Midi, I., Dogan, M., Koseoglu, M., Can, G., Sehitoglu, M., & Gunal, D. (2008). Voice abnormalities and their relation with motor dysfunction in Parkinson's disease. *Acta Neurol. Scand., 117,* 26–34.

Orozco-Arroyave, J. R., Arias-Londono, J. D., Bonilla, J. F. V., Gonzalez Rativa, M. C., & Noth, E. (2014). New Spanish speech corpus database for the analysis of people suffering from Parkinson's disease. In *International Conference on Language Resources and Evaluation* (pp. 342–347).

Rahn, D. A., Chou, M., Jiang, J. J., & Zhang, Y. (2007). Phonatory impairment in Parkinson's disease: evidence from nonlinear dynamic analysis and perturbation analysis. *J. Voice, 21,* 64–71.

Rusz, J., Cmejla, R., Ruzickova, H., & Ruzicka, E. (2011). Quantitative acoustic measurements for characterization of speech and voice disorders in early untreated Parkinson's disease. *J. Acoust. Soc. Am., 129,* 350–367.

Sakar, B. E., Isenkul, M. E., Sakar, C. O., Sertbas, A., Gurgen, F., Delil, S., Apaydin, H., & Kursun, O. (2013). Collection and analysis of a Parkinson speech dataset with multiple types of sound recordings. *IEEE J. Biomed. Health Inform., 17,* 828–834.

Shao, J., MacCallum, J. K., Zhang, Y., Sprecher, A., & Jiang, J. J. (2010). Acoustic analysis of the tremulous voice: Assessing the utility of the correlation dimension and perturbation parameters. *J. Commun. Disord., 43,* 35–44.

Simon, F., Martinez, J. P., Laguna, P., van Grinsven, B., Rutten, C., & Houben, R. (2007). Impact of sampling rate reduction on automatic ECG delineation. In *Engineering in Medicine and Biology Society, 2007. EMBS 2007. 29th Annual International Conference of the IEEE* (pp. 2587–2590). IEEE.

Ssnderson, C., & Paliwal, K. K. (1997). Effect of different sampling rates and feature vector sizes on speech recognition performance. In *TENCON'97. IEEE Region 10 Annual Conference. Speech and Image Technologies for Computing and Telecommunications., Proceedings of IEEE* (pp. 161–164). IEEE volume 1.

Stone, J. V. (2014). *Information Theory: a Tutorial Introduction.* Sheffield: Sebtel Press.

Tsanas, A. (2012). *Accurate telemonitoring of Parkinson's disease symptom severity using nonlinear speech signal processing and statistical machine learning.* Ph.D. Thesis University of Oxford.

Tsanas, A., Little, M. A., Fox, C., & Ramig, L. O. (2014a). Objective automatic assessment of rehabilitative speech treatment in Parkinson's disease. *IEEE Trans. Neural Syst. Rehabil. Eng., 22,* 181–190.

Tsanas, A., Little, M. A., McSharry, P. E., & Ramig, L. O. (2010). Enhanced classical dysphonia measures and sparse regression for telemonitoring of Parkinson's disease progression. In *Acoustics Speech and Signal Processing (ICASSP), 2010 IEEE International Conference on* (pp. 594–597). IEEE.

Tsanas, A., Little, M. A., McSharry, P. E., & Ramig, L. O. (2011). Nonlinear speech analysis algorithms mapped to a standard metric achieve clinically useful quantification of average Parkinson's disease symptom severity. *J. R. Soc. Interface., 8,* 842–855.

Tsanas, A., Little, M. A., McSharry, P. E., Spielman, J., & Ramig, L. O. (2012). Novel speech signal processing algorithms for high-accuracy classification of Parkinson's disease. *IEEE Trans. Biomed. Eng., 59,* 1264–1271.

Tsanas, A., Zaartu, M., Little, M. A., Fox, C., Ramig, L. O., & Clifford, G. D. (2014b). Robust fundamental frequency estimation in sustained vowels: detailed algorithmic comparisons and information fusion with adaptive Kalman filtering. *J. Acoust. Soc. Am., 135,* 2885–2901.

Wu, K., Zhang, D., Lu, G., & Guo, Z. (2018). Influence of sampling rate on voice analysis for assessment of Parkinson's disease. *The Journal of the Acoustical Society of America.*, *144(3)*, 1416-1423.

Zhan, A., Little, M. A., Harris, D. A., Abiola, S. O., Dorsey, E., Saria, S., & Terzis, A. (2016). High frequency remote monitoring of Parkinson's disease via smartphone: Platform overview and medication response detection. *arXiv preprint arXiv: 1601.00960.*

Chapter 3
Pitch Estimation

Abstract Pitch estimation is quite crucial to many applications. Although a number of estimation methods working in different domains have been put forward, there are still demands for improvement, especially for noisy speech. In this chapter, we present iPEEH, a general technique to raise performance of pitch estimators by enhancing harmonics. By analysis and experiments, it is found that missing and submerged harmonics are the root causes for failures of many pitch detectors. Hence, we propose to enhance the harmonics in spectrum before implementing the pitch detection. One enhancement algorithm that mainly applies the square operation to regenerate harmonics is presented in detail, including the theoretical analysis and implementation. Four speech databases with 11 types of additive noise and 5 noise levels are utilized in assessment. We compare the performance of algorithms before and after using iPEEH. Experimental results indicate that the proposed iPEEH can effectively reduce the detection errors. In some cases, the error rate reductions are higher than 20%. In addition, the advantage of iPEEH is manifold since it is demonstrated in experiments that the iPEEH is effective for various noise types, noise levels, multiple basic frequency-based estimators, and two audio types. Through this work, we investigated the underlying reasons for pitch detection failures and presented a novel direction for pitch detection. Besides, this approach, a preprocessing step in essence, indicates the significance of preprocessing for any intelligent systems.

Keywords Harmonics · Enhancement · Harmonics structure · Pitch estimation

3.1 Introduction

For voiced speech, pitch is termed as an auditory sensation of the vibration frequency of vocal cord. A high pitch means a rapid vibration, whereas a low pitch corresponds to a slow oscillation. Due to the subjectivity, researchers usually turn to use an objective scientific concept that is the fundamental frequency. In this chapter, pitch estimation refers to the detection of fundamental frequency.

© Springer Nature Singapore Pte Ltd. 2020　　　　　　　　　　　　　47
D. Zhang, K. Wu, *Pathological Voice Analysis*,
https://doi.org/10.1007/978-981-32-9196-6_3

Pitch estimation has been widely used in many speech related applications, such as speech enhancement, coding, synthesis, recognition, and speech pathology. In speech enhancement, pitch is often regarded as a useful component to reconstruct the harmonics structure that is distorted during noise suppression (Zavarehei et al. 2007). When it comes to speech coding, many systems are based on the classic source-filter model, with the source being assumed as either a white noise or a periodic signal. Hence, pitch will facilitate a correct coding of the periodic source (Spanias 1994). Similarly, the source-filter model also plays an important role in speech synthesis, which makes pitch crucial in this application (Shirota et al. 2014; Tao et al. 2006). In addition, many recognition tasks, such as the speaker recognition, emotion recognition, and speech recognition, also benefit from a precise estimated pitch. In this occasion, pitch is not only a significant discriminative feature, but also an auxiliary synchronous tool to extract other features (Kim et al. 2004). Specifically, pitch is viewed as the most important prosodic parameter for speaker recognition (Kinnunen and Li 2010; Wu and Lin 2009; Zilca et al. 2006). As to emotion and speech recognition, the role of pitch resides in its close relationship with tone (Alonso et al. 2015; Ghahremani et al. 2014; Kamaruddin et al. 2012; Rao et al. 2013; Wang et al. 2013). In speech pathology, the pitch variation for a sustained vowel, termed as jitter, is broadly applied to the diagnosis of Parkinson, vocal fold nodules, and polyps (Behroozmand et al. 2006; Das 2010; Hadjitodorov and Mitev 2002; Manfredi et al. 2000; Moran et al. 2006). Hence, pitch estimation is studied in this chapter for further pathological voice analysis.

This chapter is organized as follows. Section 3.2 reviews several frequently used pitch estimation algorithms. Section 3.3 analyzes the limitations of existing methods and introduces the proposed technique, including the theory and the implementation details. The experimental results and comparisons on pitch estimation are provided in Sect. 3.4. In Sect. 3.5, we summarize the chapter and present the future work.

3.2 Related Works

A number of algorithms have been put forward to estimate pitch. Some of them are multi-pitch estimators that are used for recordings with several speakers talking simultaneously (Christensen et al. 2008). Others are single-pitch estimators dealing with recordings with only one speaker talking. In this book, only the single-pitch case is studied. Further, methods for the single-pitch case fall into two categories: parametric and non-parametric. Generally, the parametric methods often build models based on some assumptions and then employ the maximum likelihood (ML) or maximum a posteriori (MAP) to estimate the modeling parameters (Doweck et al. 2015). As pointed out in the literature (Gonzalez and Brookes 2014), the parametric methods will be less effective if the assumptions in the modeling are not strictly satisfied. Therefore, we focus on the non-parametric algorithms only.

The available single-pitch estimation methods perform in different transform domains. In time domain, many widely used detectors are based on the correlation function or the difference function. The classic representation is the autocorrelation (ACF) approach, which estimates pitch by maximizing the ACF (Rabiner 1977). Average Magnitude Difference Function (AMDF) (Ross et al. 1974), however, is based on the difference function. By using the difference function, the multiplication operation in ACF is avoided to speed up the computation. RAPT (Talkin 1995) uses the normalized cross correlation function (NCCF) to search for the pitch candidates. To achieve a tradeoff between the computational complexity and the pitch resolution, a two-stage process is applied in the computation of NCCF. RAPT finally adopts dynamic programing as a post-processing to obtain the optimized pitch contour. YIN (De Cheveigne and Kawahara 2002) computes the squared difference function (SDF) to extract candidates, which are further refined by quadratic interpolation. This function SDF is also closely related to autocorrelation. Wautoc (Shimamura and Kobayashi 2001) is another variant that weights ACF by the inverse of AMDF. Despite the differences, these methods are all inseparably linked with ACF or AMDF.

Another common transform domain is the frequency domain. Periodicity of voiced speech is reflected as the harmonics structure in amplitude spectrum, laying the foundations for algorithms proposed in the frequency domain. For example, in Harmonic Product Spectrum algorithm (HPS) views the frequency, which maximizes the product of the spectrum at harmonics of that frequency, as the estimated pitch (Schroeder 1968). One weakness of HPS is that any missing harmonics will lead the product to be zero and then pitch detection fails (Camacho and Harris 2008). Therefore, HPS has a strong demand for an ideal harmonics structure, even for a clean speech. Subharmonic to Harmonic Ratio algorithm (SHRP) proposed by Sun (Sun 2002a) is another pitch detection algorithm in the frequency domain. In SHRP, not only the harmonics but also the subharmonics in spectrum are examined for the estimation. The subharmonics here are defined as the middle points between adjacent harmonics. The objective function in SHRP adds the spectrum at harmonics and subtracts those at the subharmonics. Note that the spectrum is transformed to logarithmic scale. It was demonstrated in SHRP that the consideration of subharmonics effects could bring some improvements.

Pitch Estimation Filter with Amplitude Compression (PEFAC) also operates in the frequency domain (Gonzalez and Brookes 2014). It convolves its spectrum with a set of filters and the one-to-one correspondences between these filters and pitch candidates are built. Since our proposed algorithm is compared with the PEFAC method in the experiment section, we show its detailed steps in the following.

Step 1. *Spectral normalization*:compute time-frequency power spectrum for each frame and normalize it using the time-averaged power spectrum.

Step 2. *Spectrum filtering*: to exploit the harmonics structure whose peaks are broadened due to the influences of window length and other factors, the filters used for PEFAC are specially designed, with their impulse responses having broadened peaks instead of the traditional delta sequence. Moreover, each of the filters comprises both positive and negative regions so that noise with a smoothly varying spectrum can be suppressed. The filter definition is as follows, where parameter γ controls the peak width and β is chosen so that $\int h(q)dq = 0$.

$$h(q) = \frac{1}{\gamma - \cos{(2\pi e^q)}} - \beta$$

Step 3. *Candidates selection*: based on the filtered spectrum, select the three highest peaks in the feasible range as pitch candidates.

Step 4. *Estimation of voice speech probability*: estimate the probability of being voiced and unvoiced with the two Gaussian mixture models (GMMs), which are trained based on normalized time-frame spectrum and the sum of the highest three peaks in the filtered spectrum.

Step 5. *Temporal continuity constraints*: adopt dynamic programming to select the sequence of candidates, in which the cost function is a weighted sum of three parameters: relative amplitude of the peaks, the rate of change of the fundamental frequency, and the deviation from the median pitch.

In this algorithm, two types of prior information are considered. One is the broadened harmonic peaks in practice and the other is the temporal continuity constraint (shown in the dynamic programming). Similarly, the BaNa algorithm (Yang et al. 2014) also considers these priors. For comparison in Sect. 3.4, the detailed steps of BaNa are given below.

Step 1. *Preprocessing*: first, the speech signal was processed with a bandpass filter, whose lower and upper bound are set to F_0^{min} and $p \times F_0^{max}$, respectively. Here F_0^{min} and F_0^{max} are the lower and upper limit and of fundamental frequency of human speech, respectively. p is a parameter to be set, denoting the number of spectral peaks captured.

Step 2. *Determination of F0 candidates:* F0 candidates are generated based on the assumption that harmonics are regularly spaced at approximately integer multiples of the fundamental frequency in the frequency domain. After the preprocessing in Step 1, frequencies with high peaks are selected from the spectrum. Then these frequencies are sorted in an ascending order and ratios between any two of them (the higher to the lower) are calculated. If a calculated ratio falls into any predefined tolerance ranges, one pitch candidate is generated accordingly. All ratios perform in the same way and a set of pitch candidates are generated. Besides, pitch derived from the cepstrum method (Noll 1967) is added to the set, too. Candidates here are then clustered to form a smaller set. In this new set, each candidate is given a confidence score defined as the number of its close candidates during merging.

Step 3. *Selection of F0 from candidates*: eventually, a global pitch track optimization across all frames is gained by Viterbi algorithm, where the total cost considers both the frequency consistence between two consecutive frames and the confidence score for each candidate. The last step gives this algorithm more noise resilience.

In BaNa, the tolerance ranges are designed to deal with the broadening of harmonic peaks as in the PEFAC and Viterbi works on the assumption of temporal continuity, resembling the dynamic programming in PEFAC. As is seen, a majority of algorithms in this domain use spectrum in a direct way without any modification or enhancement.

Other useful domains for pitch extraction include the wavelet domain (Chen and Wang 2002; Ercelebi 2003) and the Hilbert–Huang domain (Huang and Pan 2006). Recently, data-driven statistical approaches are increasingly popular. One typical algorithm TAPS (Temporally Accumulated Peaks Spectrum) is presented by Huang and Lee (2013). It is based on the observation that the harmonics structure of speech often holds slower change than the noise spectrum so that an accumulation operation can suppress noise to a lower level. Therefore, the accumulated peaks spectrum will be robust against noise. After the accumulation, pitch is estimated by sparse representation of TAPS and the dictionary used is trained using clean speeches. Another statistical method is the work of Han and Wang (2014). Kun Han used two neural networks, deep neural networks (DNNs) and recurrent neural networks (RNNs), to model the pitch state distribution by treating the noisy frames as observations. In the end, Viterbi decoding follows to form the continuous pitch contour. Specifically, the features used are captured in the spectral domain and noisy speeches of different noise types and noise levels compose the training set. Despite the great performance, these data-driven approaches may be infeasible in practice due to their limited generalization. Usually, the training set is closely related to the test set so that the learned model must be retrained in a new acoustic environment with a new training set. However, the matched training set is not always available. In a word, data-driven approaches often possess generalization problem.

Despite all these works, two considerations have motivated us to investigate the same topic further. Firstly, the computational complexities of many algorithms performing well for noisy speeches are often high and their computational speeds are unsatisfying. For these high-speed methods, however, their performances often degrade greatly when the speeches are contaminated by noise. Thus, as Yang et al. (2014) have pointed out, pitch estimation for noisy speeches is still a challenging issue and there is still large room for improvement. One may doubt that noise in the noisy speeches can be removed by noise suppression algorithms and there is no need to study the pitch estimation for noisy speech. Here it is worthwhile to mention that the estimated pitch also plays a key role for speech enhancement. Hence, detecting pitch for noisy speeches is quite necessary in practice. Secondly, the main types of errors for many pitch estimation algorithms can be summarized as the harmonic errors and the subharmonic errors. To solve this issue, one common way is to apply the global optimization, assuming that pitches for adjacent frames do not vary much. However, in some applications, pitch must be estimated for each frame independently. For instance, pitch for the pathological speech may vary dramatically, even in the local regions. In this case, the valuable pathological information will be lost if global optimization is applied. Hence, pitch estimation with great performance for individual frame is in great demand. Based on these two considerations, further research on this topic is needed.

Noise affects the estimation of pitch by degrading the periodicity in speech. Under extreme conditions, such as when the signal-to-noise ratio (SNR) drops down to negative dB, the periodicity can be destroyed and unrecoverable. In our book, severely corrupted noisy speech is beyond our research and we focus on the noisy speeches with a global SNR from 0 dB to 20 dB. Additionally, only one speaker is speaking in each of the recordings, meaning that we are studying the single-pitch estimation problem only. In addition, the voiced/unvoiced determination is another inevitable consideration for pitch detection since pitch is only meaningful for the voiced frames. While some existing works have investigated the voicing detection and pitch estimation together (Gonzalez and Brookes 2014; Han and Wang 2014; Sun 2002a), other have treated them separately (De Cheveigne and Kawahara 2002; Huang and Lee 2013; Yang et al. 2014). For the latter case, these methods assume that the voicing state for each frame has been correctly decided before and pitch estimation is then applied to the voiced frames only. Thus, methods are evaluated on databases whose voiced/unvoiced decisions have been made. Similarly, we consider the pitch estimation only and the voiced/unvoiced detection is not within the scope of this chapter. Instead of putting forward an independent pitch detector, we propose a universal technique, by which the performance of common frequency-based algorithms can be raised. As introduced, pitch estimators cover several different domains and frequency domain is chosen in our method due to its excellent properties. Firstly, the spectrum of voiced speech is often shown as multiple impulses-like peaks. Secondly, the peaks are approximately linearly spaced. Those two outstanding features can ease the pattern modeling. Thirdly, for speech corrupted by narrow banded noise, the effect of noise is only concentrated on limited sub-bands. Estimators operating in spectrum are more advantageous in this case. Therefore, we focus on estimating pitch in the frequency domain. To improve the performance, we firstly examine the existing approaches in this domain and analyze their common limitations: bad harmonics structure. Then we are motivated to enhance the spectrum before using it in estimation and a well-performed harmonics enhancement strategy is presented in detail. The proposed technique is named as iPEEH. Finally, experiments show that the iPEEH can partially overcome the limitations of many previous works and pitch detection by applying the proposed technique achieves lower error rates. Besides, the experimental results also demonstrate the generality of iPEEH since it is effective for multiple noise types, noise levels, and four types of original algorithms. Moreover, pitch estimation for music resembles that for speech. Therefore, this technique is also extended to the pitch detection of music. Note that emphasis in this chapter is on the pitch detection for voiced speech and the application for music is just covered as an example to demonstrate the generality of the proposed technique.

3.3 Harmonics Enhancement for Pitch Estimation

3.3.1 Motivation for Harmonics Enhancement

Many pitch detection algorithms working in the frequency domain are established on the harmonics structure of spectrum. This spectrum is assumed to show spikes at harmonics and amplitudes at frequencies other than the harmonics are supposed to be lower. In an ideal condition, a frame of speech is strictly periodic and its spectrum amplitude equals to zero everywhere except at harmonics. Hence, it is reasonable to assume that a perfect harmonics structure, being suitable for pitch detection, is inclined to be significant at harmonics and inconspicuous at others. Here we term a spectrum with such harmonics structure as an ideal spectrum.

However, many factors will result in destructions of this ideal structure. Speech is produced under the cooperation of multiple organs, including lung, vocal cords, and vocal tract. In the classical source-filter model, the vibration of vocal cords generates the source for the voiced speeches and the tract acts as the filter. Ideally, the source of the voiced speech is an impulse train in time domain and its Fourier transform is exactly another impulse train. Owning to the vocal tract, the filter, the speech spectrum is then characterized with formants and the amplitudes at harmonics differ greatly. In extreme case, some harmonics disappear even for a clean speech frame. As pointed by Camacho and Harris (2008), one of the failure reasons for HPS is due to the missing harmonics. As a result, pitch detection for a clean speech may also fail. For a noisy speech, harmonics with smaller amplitude are likely to be submerged by the noise around. In conclusion, both the vocal tract and the external noise can bring damages to the ideal harmonics structure and these damages are shown as missing or submerged harmonics. As mentioned in the last paragraph, the ideal spectrum is the one suitable for estimation. Thus, we state that these factors doing damage to the ideal harmonics structure are also the reasons for a pitch detection failure.

An ideal spectrum with good harmonics structure is the key for the pitch estimation. However, as what has been introduced in Sect. 3.1, the existing algorithms often operate directly on a spectrum without considering the quality of its harmonics structure. To overcome the limitations in the current research, it is essential to reconstruct the harmonics structure before using it in estimation. Actually, a strategy named as harmonics enhancement or harmonics regeneration can fulfill this demand and the enhanced harmonics structure should then show relatively distinct peaks at harmonics and low values at other locations. Currently, the strategy of harmonics enhancement is mainly adopted in two applications. One application is the speech enhancement, in which the harmonics enhancement is to post process the speech signal after noise reduction so that the distorted harmonics can be enhanced (Plapous et al. 2005; Jin et al. 2010). The other is in the speech separation application and the harmonics in spectral are enhanced to separate the desired speaker (Bouafif and Lachiri 2014; Krishnamoorthy and Prasanna 2010).

The harmonics enhancement presented here is often confused with the speech enhancement. Thus, it is worthwhile to make a comparison between the harmonics enhancement and the speech enhancement. Firstly, harmonics enhancement here is designed to improve the pitch estimation performance, whereas speech enhancement is used to remove noise. Secondly, speech enhancement is applied to noisy speeches only, while harmonics enhancement is applicable to both clean and noisy speeches. Thirdly, one critical evaluation metric for speech enhancement is the distortion rate, which is computed by comparing the enhanced speeches with the reference clean speeches. However, there is no reference for harmonics enhancement. Fourthly, speech enhancement is to remove the unwanted noise while keeping the signal unchanged. Conversely, harmonics enhancement attempts to improve the harmonics structure, regardless of the changes introduced to the speech (but change to the pitch is not allowed). Finally, speech enhancement often acts as a role of preprocessing for many speech-related applications and the enhanced speech may be repeatedly used. Nevertheless, harmonics enhancement here is used for pitch detection only and the enhanced harmonics structure will not be used elsewhere. Through this comparison, it can be derived that harmonics enhancement is quite another topic and the proposed approach in this chapter may not be suitable for speech enhancement.

3.3.2 Theoretical Analysis

In this part, we provide the theoretical analysis for the proposed method. The analysis here is performed in the time domain and speech frame is assumed strictly periodic during the analysis.

After frame division, each frame of the voiced speech can be analyzed by the Fourier transform. Since the speech frame is periodic under ideal condition, Fourier series is then used to decompose the frame signal into a superimposition of several sines and cosines. Ideally, frequencies for these sines (cosines) are integer multiple of the fundamental frequency, which are termed as harmonics. Hence, in complex form of Fourier series, the speech can be represented by the following equation.

$$f(t) = \sum_{n=-\infty}^{\infty} c_n e^{j2\pi n f_0 t} \tag{3.1}$$

Here $f(t)$ is the frame signal. Parameter f_0 is the fundamental frequency and the coefficient c_n, generally a complex number, is called Fourier coefficient. j in Eq. (3.1) stands for the imaginary unit. For simplicity, we analyze a simple case when the speech is composed of two harmonics only and then the signal can be written as

$$f_1(t) = c_m e^{j2\pi m f_0 t} + c_k e^{j2\pi k f_0 t}, \quad k \in Z \text{ and } m \in Z \tag{3.2}$$

where the term $e^{j2\pi m f_0 t}$ indicates the mth harmonic. According to the property of exponential function, the following equality holds.

$$\left(c_m e^{j2\pi m f_0 t}\right) * \left(c_k e^{j2\pi k f_0 t}\right) = c_m c_k e^{j2\pi(m+k) f_0 t} \tag{3.3}$$

It is evident that a new harmonic can be regenerated through a multiplication of two existing harmonics. It indicates that some missing harmonics can be regenerated by proper manipulation operations. In fact, this observation inspires the core of the proposed method.

Motivated by the above analysis, we intend to square the speech. The square operation is chosen since it brings all pairwise products of the existing harmonics. Then $f_1^2(t)$ can be expressed as follows.

$$f_1^2(t) = c_m^2 e^{j2\pi(2m)f_0 t} + c_k^2 e^{j2\pi(2k)f_0 t} + 2c_m c_k e^{j2\pi(m+k)f_0 t} \qquad (3.4)$$

Here, we can see this calculation results in three new harmonics: $(2m)$th, $(2k)$th, and $(m + k)$th (these three harmonics may overlap). Two harmonics here $((2m)$th and $(2k)$th) are twice of the harmonics in the original signal (mth and kth). The other harmonic $(m + k)$th is the addition result. Usually, the three harmonics in Eq. (3.3) are not included in the original signal $f_1(t)$. In other words, this calculation generates new harmonics. Actually, this transformation is the core for our algorithm. A simple example is given for better understanding. Assume that m is 2 and k equals to 3, then the squared signal can be expressed as

$$f_1^2(t) = c_2^2 e^{j2\pi 4 f_0 t} + c_3^2 e^{j2\pi 6 f_0 t} + 2c_2 c_3 e^{j2\pi 5 f_0 t} \qquad (3.5)$$

Clearly, the original speech $f_1(t)$ contains two harmonics (second and third), whereas the newly squared signal $f_1^2(t)$ includes three new harmonics (fourth, fifth, and sixth). Besides, adding $f_1(t)$ with $f_1^2(t)$ can further extend the harmonic number and the sum has five harmonics altogether. In this example, two steps are critical. Firstly, the square operation is adopted to generate new harmonics. Secondly, to replenish the harmonic structure, the squared signal is further added to the original signal. In fact, these two steps have increase the number of harmonics, implying that the harmonics structure is enhanced.

The simplified case above, consisting of two harmonics only, can be generalized to a more complex occasion. When more harmonics are involved, square operation remains applicable to generate new harmonics. It can be easily proved that the square operation results in the following harmonics: twice of the original harmonics and the addition of any two harmonics in the original signal. Therefore, adding the squared speech to the original speech can enrich the harmonics structure, just as what has been shown in the simplified example.

Our proposed approach is based on the above analysis and the basic idea can be summarized as adding the squared signal to the original one. Since the aim is to enhance the harmonics structure, we explain how the enhancement works in detail. The role of enhancement is two-folds. First, the square operation has produced new harmonics, some of which may be not contained in the original signal. In other words, the squared signal covers fresh harmonics. In this sense, the proposed mechanism enables the filling of absent harmonics. Secondly, if there are intersections between the newly derived harmonics set and that of the original signal, then the enhancement brings in amplitude increase for the overlapped harmonics. In summing up of these two aspects, the proposed technique has the function of number filling, or amplitude enhancement, or both. Thus, using the operations of square and addition, the harmonics structure can be enhanced, either in terms of number or the amplitude.

3.3.3 Implementation

In Sect. 3.3.2, we have analyzed the harmonics enhancement under an ideal assumption that speech is strictly periodic. However, speech frame in practice, even for the steady clean speech, is not strictly periodic and the harmonics are not always integer multiples of the fundamental frequency. Here, we claim that the proposed theory can be extended to a real speech. Actually, the key for the proposed method lies in Eq. (3.3). When the parameters m and k in this equation are not strictly integers, this equation still holds. Thus, new harmonics can also be generated through the square operation and speech in real case can apply this method.

For the enhancement performed in practice, a few more steps are needed. A schematic diagram of the multistage steps is shown in Fig. 3.1. Each step is expounded explicitly as follows. Figure 3.2 is added to illustrate this method by applying it to a voiced frame. This frame comes from a noisy speech mixed by the babble noise from NOISEX-92 noise database (Varga et al. 1992) and a clean speech in KEELE database (Plante et al. 1995). The global SNR for this noisy speech is 5 dB.

3.3.3.1 Enframe and FFT

The enframe operation is to divide the speech signal into frames and FFT is then used to obtain the absolute amplitude spectrum. Here, the window type, frame length, inter-frame time increment, and FFT length are chosen accordingly. In the presented example in Fig. 3.2, the window type is the Hann window. The frame length and inter-frame time increment are set as 60 ms and 10 ms, respectively. Besides, the FFT length is assigned as 2^{16} (the sampling rate is 16,000 Hz).

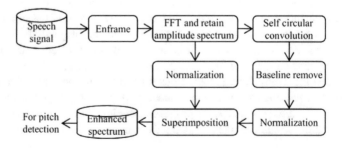

Fig. 3.1 Schematic diagram of the proposed enhancement method

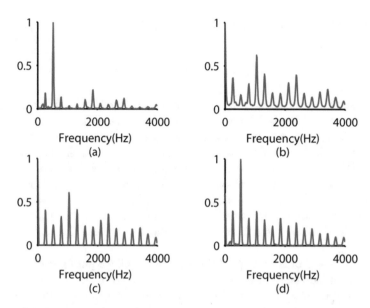

Fig. 3.2 Illustration of harmonics enhancement using the proposed method on a frame of voiced noisy speech. (**a**) The original spectrum. (**b**) Self-circular convolution result. (**c**) Spectrum after removing the baseline in (**b**). (**d**) Final enhanced spectrum

3.3.3.2 Self-Circular Convolution

Square is used for the enhancement in Sect. 3.3.2. However, it is noteworthy that there is a major defect for the square. Although the square operation brings new harmonics, the amplitudes for these harmonics are often unsatisfying. Therefore, harmonics enhancement in this way may be not effective.

To understand the reason behind, a brief explanation is provided here. Representing the real speech using Eq. (3.1), then the absolute amplitude for hth harmonic in the squared signal will equal to

$$\begin{cases} \left| \left(c_{h/2} \right)^2 + 2 \sum_{i=-\infty}^{\infty} c_i c_{h-i} \right|, & \text{if } h \text{ is even} \\ 2 \left| \sum_{i=-\infty}^{\infty} c_i c_{h-i} \right|, & \text{if } h \text{ is odd.} \end{cases} \tag{3.6}$$

Here ‖ means a modulus operator. In this equation, the harmonic amplitude is a sum of many product terms and each term is the multiplication of two variables c_i and c_{h-i}. Since the coefficients c_i and c_{h-i} are complex numbers, the product terms are also complex numbers. Therefore, the amplitude of the harmonic is the absolute value of the sum of many complex numbers. However, this direct sum of complex numbers cannot achieve the maximum amplitude and this is one underlying reason for the indistinctive harmonic amplitude. To prove this statement, the well-known triangle inequality concerning modulus of complex numbers is presented below (Stillwell 2005).

$$| C_1 + C_2 | \leq | C_1 | + | C_2 | \tag{3.7}$$

Here C_1 and C_2 are any two complex numbers. This inequality is still true when the number of terms in the sum increases. According to this inequality, the summation result in Eq. (3.6) is not the optimum result and the harmonic amplitude can be improved. In addition, the equality in the above inequality holds if and only if $C_1 = 0$ or $C_2 = 0$, or $C_2 = \alpha C_1$ for some $\alpha > 0$. Similarly, the multiple product terms in Eq. (3.6) must share the same phase so that the equality holds. However, this condition is quite strict and the product terms rarely meet this demand. Hence, the harmonics amplitudes for the squared speech are likely to be low and indistinct. This partially explains why the harmonics amplitudes for the squared speech are unsatisfying.

To remedy this disadvantage of the squared signal, we put forward to raise the amplitudes of harmonics in the squared speech. The basic principle is to make the equality in Eq. (3.7) hold. In detail, the coefficients c_i and c_{h-i} in Eq. (3.6) are replaced with their absolute values. Namely, the phases for all the complex coefficients are assigned with the same value 0. In this way, the product terms in Eq. (3.6) share the same phase and the equality in Eq. (3.7) holds. Thus, maximum amplitudes are achieved. In consequence, the maximized amplitude for the hth harmonic is

$$\begin{cases} \left(|c_{h/2}|\right)^2 + 2 \sum\limits_{i=-\infty}^{\infty} | c_i \| c_{h-i} | , & \text{if } h \text{ is even} \\ 2 \sum\limits_{i=-\infty}^{\infty} | c_i \| c_{h-i} | , & \text{if } h \text{ is odd.} \end{cases} \tag{3.8}$$

To sum up, the remedy works by modifying the signal before square operation and the modification is to unify the phase of Fourier coefficients as 0.

With respect to detailed implementation, this enhancement is performed in the frequency domain. Firstly, the absolute amplitude spectrum is obtained using FFT. The amplitudes here are non-negative real values and the phase information is ignored (all phases are set to 0). Secondly, according to the convolution theorem, the square operation in time domain is realized by the self-circular convolution of the absolute amplitude spectrum. Hereafter, the newly method resulting Eq. (3.8) is called the *convolution method,* while the enhancement using a direct square without abandoning the phase information is named as the *square method.* Other remaining steps are kept the same for these two methods.

The circular convolution result for the spectrum in Fig. 3.2a is shown in Fig. 3.2b. Many unclear harmonics in Fig. 3.2a appear clearly in Fig. 3.2b, especially those in the high frequency zone. Besides, the baseline wander is obvious.

3.3.3.3   Baseline Removal

The spectrum after convolution has a baseline wander. Therefore, baseline removal is needed. Observation shows that the baseline changes more slowly than the harmonic peaks. Therefore, it is proposed to remove the baseline wander by a high-pass filter. For this filtering, the current spectrum is firstly transformed using FFT. Then the coefficients corresponding to frequencies lower than the cut-off frequency (11 Hz) are simply assigned to zero. Finally, the inverse Fourier transform is carried out. This filtering technique removes the baseline wander. Besides, the high-pass filter has made the amplitudes in the filtered result to fluctuate around 0. Then amplitudes with negative values are assigned to zero, which is in fact a noise flooring technique (Jin et al. 2010). Using this method to spectrum in Fig. 3.2b, the baseline is removed as exhibited in Fig. 3.2c. In fact, the noise flooring technique used here can reduce influence of noise and it is evident in Fig. 3.2c that the amplitudes for the non-harmonics are lower and indistinctive.

3.3.3.4   Spectrum Superimposition

Just as the simplified example in Sect. 3.3.2, the spectrum after convolution may not contain the harmonics of original spectrum. Therefore, the two spectrums are added together to increase the robustness of enhancement. Before addition, each of them is normalized by its own Euclidean norm. Figure 3.2d displays the result of superimposition. Comparing with the spectrum in Fig. 3.2c, the amplitude of the second harmonic is greatly improved. In the original spectrum, there is only one distinct peak. Apart from this harmonic, most harmonics are missing or submerged by the ambient noise. The enhanced spectrum in Fig. 3.2d, however, shows great improvement since most of the harmonics display distinct amplitudes and they can be easily discriminated from the noise around. In fact, the enhancement is shown in two aspects: the gain of harmonics amplitudes and the increase of harmonics number. For the pitch estimation, spectrum in Fig. 3.2d is preferred to that in Fig. 3.2a and the scientific comparisons are implemented in Sect. 3.4.

3.3.3.5   Usage in Pitch Estimation

The enhanced spectrum has filled the missing or destroyed harmonics, making it more suitable for pitch estimation than the original spectrum. In this section, the use of the enhanced spectrum during pitch estimation is provided. For simplicity, the proposed method is abbreviated as iPEEH (Improving Pitch Estimation by Enhancing Harmonics). Note that the enhancement in iPEEH applies the convolution method and iPEEH is applied to the frequency-based pitch estimation methods only.

The usage is straightforward and simple. Frequency-based approaches use the spectrum of each frame. Before using the spectrum, iPEEH is employed to enhance it and the enhanced spectrum is used thereafter. Other than this replacement, the pitch estimation algorithms remain unchanged. Namely, the usage of iPEEH is to replace the original spectrum with the enhanced spectrum. Obviously, this modification is easy to implement. In addition, the high expansibility is apparent since any frequency-based estimators can apply our method.

3.3.4 In-Depth Analysis of the Proposed Algorithm

In this section, two preliminary experiments are displayed. One is designed to demonstrate that harmonics structure is vital for pitch estimation. The other experiment shows that the proposed method can significantly improve the harmonics structure. Based on these two results, the feasibility of the proposed iPEEH is testified. At the end of this section, the time complexity of iPEEH is analyzed.

3.3.4.1 Harmonics Structure and Pitch Estimation

Harmonics structure plays an important role in pitch estimation. In this part, an experiment is presented to show the importance.

To describe the harmonics structure objectively, a metric HNR (harmonics to noise ratio) is adopted. Generally, HNR is commonly used as a feature to identify pathological speech (Qi and Hillman 1997; Kasuya et al. 1986; Naranjo et al. 2016; Yumoto et al. 1982) and the nature of HNR is to compute the energy ratio of the harmonics portion to the noise portion. Thus, we adopt this metric to measure the quality of the harmonics structure. Generally, an ideal harmonics structure has a high HNR and any damages to the ideal harmonics structure cause a decline of HNR. For a clean frame, if some harmonics are missing, then the harmonics quantity is reduced and so is the corresponding HNR. Likewise, corrupting noise increases the noise amount, leading to a reduction of the HNR. Therefore, it is reasonable to apply the HNR as an objective metric to interpret.

Through the above analysis, it can be claimed that a spectrum with a high HNR is more suitable for estimating pitch, whereas a low HNR often leads to detection errors in frequency-based pitch detection algorithms.

To convince this declaration, an experimental result is provided to show the relationship between HNR and the estimation accuracy. For a given recording, all voiced frames are marked in advance. Then these marked frames are divided into two classes by adopting a spectrum-based pitch estimation method HPS, which has been introduced in Sect. 3.1. One class includes frames with correctly estimated pitches and the other is for frames with incorrectly detected pitches. For clarity, these two classes are named as *class A* and *class B*, respectively. According to our analysis, the harmonics structure in *class A* should be better than that in *class B*. Thus, this experiment aims to compare the average HNRs of these two classes.

Some basic experiment settings are described here. Firstly, the adopted recording dataset consists of noisy speeches, which are mixed by clean speeches and noise. Noise types include babble noise (*N1*), destroyer engine room noise (*N2*), destroyer operations room noise (*N3*), factory floor noise (*N4*), high frequency radio channel noise (*N5*), pink noise(*N6*), vehicle interior noise (*N7*), white noise (*N8*), tank noise (*N9*), military vehicle noise(*N10*), and F-16 cockpit noise(*N11*). These pure noises are from the NOISEX-92 noise database (Varga et al. 1992). SNRs are in five levels: 0 dB, 5 dB, 10 dB, 15 dB, and 20 dB. Besides, ten clean speeches in the KEELE database (Plante et al. 1995) are used. With all the combinations, there are 550 recordings altogether. Each recording here sustains as long as around 30 s so that the frame numbers for *class A* and *class B* in each recording are large enough for statistics. Secondly, the estimated pitch is counted as incorrect if the detected pitch deviates more than 10% from its ground truth. In addition, the ground truth pitches mentioned here are available online (Ba et al. 2013) and these true values are actually calculated on the simultaneously recorded laryngograph signals. Thirdly, the actual HNR definition used in this experiment is presented. For each frame,

$$\text{HNR} = 20\log \frac{\sum_{n=1}^{M} \sum_{\delta=-0.1f_0}^{0.1f_0} S(nf_0 + \delta)}{\sum S - \sum_{n=1}^{M} \sum_{\delta=-0.1f_0}^{0.1f_0} S(nf_0 + \delta)} \qquad (3.9)$$

Here S is the amplitude spectrum and f_0 is the ground truth fundamental frequency. For the parameter M, it is set as the maximum integer that meets $M \times f_0 \leq 3500$, assuming that there is no obvious harmonics higher than 3500 Hz. Every harmonic region is set by an interval of $\pm 0.1f_0$. This interval is set due to the broadening of the harmonics peaks as pointed out by Gonzalez and Brookes (2014). The unit of HNR is dB. This definition is simplified and it is not strictly accurate since the amplitudes at harmonics are in fact the combined effect of harmonics and noise. In the definition here, however, noise is restricted beyond harmonic regions. Therefore, the real HNR should be smaller than that in this definition. Since the HNR defined here is used to implement comparisons, the exact choice of the interval width does not matter much and the simplification of HNR definition is acceptable. Fourthly, the window type, frame length, inter-frame time increment, and FFT length are the same as in Sect. 3.3.3.1.

In the experiment, two average HNRs are computed for each recording. They are obtained by averaging HNRs over frames in *class A* and *class B,* respectively. Then the difference of the two HNRs is calculated. Thus, in this database, there are 550 differences. According to the analysis before, all of these differences should be positive. Here the distribution of these 550 differences is shown in Fig. 3.3. The distribution is relatively concentrated and all of the 550 differences are greater than 0. This statistical result confirms that a good harmonics structure indicated by a high HNR is more suitable for pitch estimation.

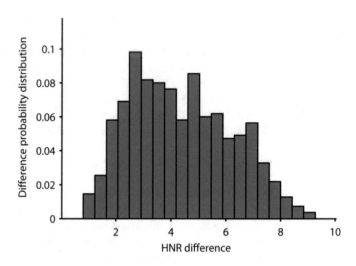

Fig. 3.3 Distribution of the HNR difference

Through this experiment, two conclusions are drawn. In the first place, HNR is one proper metric to measure the quality of harmonics structure. Secondly, the harmonics structure is crucial for pitch estimation and bad harmonics structure (low HNR) is one reason for the pitch estimation failure.

In case of spectrum with a low HNR, the previous studies work directly on this spectrum without attempt to improve the structure. In our chapter, we have proposed the iPEEH to enhance the harmonics structure before estimation so that the pitch detection rate can be raised.

3.3.4.2   Feasibility Analysis

As analyzed, one reason for the pitch detection error is the low HNR. iPEEH is proposed to enhance the harmonics for the purpose of increasing the HNR. In this part, we validate that whether the proposed harmonics enhancement method boosts the HNR.

For the validation, three classes of HNRs are compared. One is the HNR calculated based on the original spectrum, providing the baseline for comparison. The second HNR is computed using the spectrum enhanced by the *square method*. In Sect. 3.3, we have concluded that there is a big weakness of the direct *square method* when enhancing harmonics and there is still large room for improvement. Thus, this HNR is added to testify this conclusion. The last HNR adopts the spectrum enhanced by the *convolution method*. For each voiced frame in a recording, the three HNRs are calculated, which are denoted as $fHNR^{(orig)}$, $fHNR^{(square)}$, and $fHNR^{(conv)}$, respectively.

For the basic experimental set, it is similar to that in Sect. 3.3.1. This set contains 550 noisy speech recordings of 11 noise types and 5 SNR levels. In this experiment, this set is divided into 55 subsets. In each subset, the noisy speeches are corrupted by the same noise type and noise level. Finally, three averaged HNRs for each subset, which are $c\text{HNR}^{(\text{orig})}$, $c\text{HNR}^{(\text{square})}$, and $c\text{HNR}^{(\text{conv})}$, are presented. In detail, the averages are calculated by

$$c\text{HNR}^{(eAL)} = \frac{1}{SE} \sum_{i=1}^{SE} \left(\frac{1}{F_i} \sum_{j=1}^{F_i} f\text{HNR}_{ij}^{(eAL)} \right);$$

$$eAL \in \{\text{orig}, \text{square}, \text{conv}\}$$

(3.10)

where F_i is the voiced frame number of the ith noisy speech in the current subset and SE represents the number of noisy speeches in this subset. In our experiment, SE equals to 10. Parameter $f\text{HNR}_{ij}^{(eAL)}$ is the HNR for the jth voiced frame in the ith noisy speech by adopting the enhancement algorithm specified by eAL.

Therefore, for each method, 55 average HNRs are acquired, corresponding to all possible combinations of noise type and SNR level. As shown in Table 3.1, the *square method* can improve HNR comparing with the HNR computed on the original spectrum in most cases, with an exception of the m109 noise at 0 dB. However, HNRs using the *convolution method* are higher than HNRs of the original spectrum for all cases. In addition, the comparison also discloses the performance difference of the *square method* and the *convolution method*. For all cases, HNRs for the *convolution method* are higher than that for the *square method*. Finally, the overall HNR improvements by those two methods are shown in Table 3.2. Here the HNR improvement by the *convolution method* is about 1.5 dB higher than that by the *square method*. Based on the comparisons, we conclude that both the *square* and *convolution method* can improve the HNR, indicating an enhancement of the harmonics structure. Besides, the *square method* is inferior to the *convolution method* in terms of HNR improvement. These results are in consistent with the analysis in Sect. 3.2.

The experimental result implies that the proposed *convolution method* can increase the HNR values effectively, indicating the improvement of harmonics structure. As concluded in Sect. 3.3.1, a better harmonics structure suggests less detection errors. Thus, the feasibility of iPEEH is verified.

3.3.4.3 Speeding Up Strategy and Time Complexity Analysis

For the enhancement, there is room for further optimization to reduce the running time. We notice that the self-circular convolution in Sect. 3.3.3 is the most time consuming step. To optimize, the retained amplitude spectrum is regarded as a signal denoted as S and the self-circular convolution of the signal is realized by the square operation in its FFT domain. This process can be expressed as

Table 3.1 HNR performance for noisy speech of varied noise types and SNR levels

Noise type	Methods	0 dB	5 dB	10 dB	15 dB	20 dB
Babble (N1)	Original	−3.91	−2.16	−0.25	1.53	2.96
	Square	−3.63	−1.46	0.96	3.14	4.80
	Convolution	**−2.40**	**0.16**	**2.67**	**4.73**	**6.24**
Destroyer engine (N2)	Original	−3.97	−2.27	−0.39	1.38	2.82
	Square	−3.87	−1.80	0.56	2.76	4.50
	Convolution	**−3.19**	**−0.69**	**1.88**	**4.12**	**5.82**
Destroyer-ops (N3)	Original	−3.71	−1.92	0.00	1.76	3.14
	Square	−3.46	−1.26	1.19	3.38	5.01
	Convolution	**−2.37**	**0.30**	**2.90**	**4.99**	**6.44**
Factory (N4)	Original	−4.31	−2.58	−0.63	1.23	2.75
	Square	−4.04	−1.92	0.52	2.81	4.59
	Convolution	**−2.79**	**−0.23**	**2.33**	**4.47**	**6.07**
Hf channel (N5)	Original	−4.48	−3.00	−1.25	0.54	2.13
	Square	−4.29	−2.45	−0.23	1.99	3.86
	Convolution	**−3.02**	**−0.82**	**1.48**	**3.60**	**5.34**
Pink (N6)	Original	−4.33	−2.59	−0.63	1.24	2.76
	Square	−3.98	−1.83	0.61	2.87	4.63
	Convolution	**−2.36**	**0.15**	**2.58**	**4.63**	**6.15**
Volvo (N7)	Original	0.48	2.10	3.31	4.13	4.64
	Square	1.69	3.51	4.91	5.89	6.50
	Convolution	**4.12**	**5.77**	**6.87**	**7.56**	**7.95**
White (N8)	Original	−3.73	−2.04	−0.20	1.53	2.94
	Square	−3.40	−1.27	1.06	3.17	4.79
	Convolution	**−1.74**	**0.64**	**2.90**	**4.81**	**6.25**
M109 (N9)	Original	−3.68	−1.64	0.38	2.10	3.39
	Square	−3.84	−1.40	1.19	3.45	5.09
	Convolution	**−3.52**	**−0.48**	**2.51**	**4.87**	**6.45**
Leopard (N10)	Original	−2.82	−1.01	0.79	2.34	3.50
	Square	−2.64	−0.35	2.01	3.99	5.39
	Convolution	**−1.61**	**1.14**	**3.65**	**5.54**	**6.78**
F16 (N11)	Original	−4.54	−2.84	−0.90	0.99	2.57
	Square	−4.33	−2.24	0.21	2.54	4.39
	Convolution	**−3.16**	**−0.60**	**1.98**	**4.20**	**5.87**

Bold values indicate better results

Table 3.2 Overall HNR improvement (dB) for different methods

Methods	Square	Convolution
Overall average HNR improvement(dB)	1.10	**2.62**

Bold values indicate better results

$$S * S = C \cdot \mathscr{F}^{-1}\left\{\mathscr{F}\{S\}^2\right\} \tag{3.11}$$

where $\mathscr{F}\{S\}$ denotes the Fourier transform of S, $\mathscr{F}^{-1}$ is the inverse Fourier transform, and C is a constant. Besides, the baseline removal in Sect. 3.3.3 is implemented in the frequency domain of $S * S$. Thus, after the square operation on the right side of Eq. (3.11), we do not finish the inverse Fourier transform immediately, but choose to perform the baseline removal in this domain directly. That is to assign the coefficients in $\mathscr{F}\{S\}^2$ corresponding to frequencies lower than the cut-off frequency (11 Hz) to zero. Finally, the inverse Fourier transform is applied. By this way, the main computations are realized by a FFT transform and an inverse FFT transform.

After the optimized implementation, time complexity analysis of the enhancement is provided here. For each frame, we assume that the FFT length used is N. Then the time complexity to compute the absolute amplitude spectrum is O (N log N). The time complexity to finish the self-circular convolution and the baseline removal is also O(N log N). Finally, the superimposition together with the needed normalizations has a time complexity of O(N). Hence, it is obvious that the running time in each step depends on the FFT length.

3.4   Experimental Result

Since the proposed iPEEH holds universality, four popular pitch estimation methods, HPS (Schroeder 1968), SHRP (Sun 2002b), PEFAC (Gonzalez and Brookes 2014), and BaNa (Yang et al. 2014), working in the frequency domain are embedded with the iPEEH. All of them share a similarity that they estimate pitch from the spectrum in a direct way while no improvement or modification to the spectrum is applied. Applying the usage presented in Sect. 3.3.3, the proposed iPEEH is embedded into each of the four methods to form the embedded methods which are named by adding prefix "im" to their original names, i.e., imHPS, imSHRP, imPEFAC, and imBaNa.

Note that the differences among the four original methods are outside our concern and we focus on the performance improvement of each method after applying iPEEH. More detail about this section, such as experimental setting and results, are well demonstrated in literature (Wu et al. 2016).

3.4.1   Basic Experimental Setting

The noisy speeches used in our experiments are generated by mixing the clean speeches with noise. The clean speech datasets come from four sources (Yang et al. 2014): LDC, Arctic, CSTR, and KEELE. For more detailed information on the databases, one can refer to the literature (Yang et al. 2014). For the pure noise, we adopt the same noise types (11 in total) and levels (5 in total) as in Sect. 3.3. In addition, we focus on the pitch estimation only in this chapter and strategy in a previous work (Yang et al. 2014) was adopted for voicing detection. As for the performance evaluation, we adopt the Gross Pitch Error (GPE) rate as the metric, in which if the deviation exceeds 10% of the ground truth pitch, this detection is counted as a Gross Pitch Error.

The proposed harmonics enhancement is carried out on a single frame. For fair comparison, the post processing in both PEFAC and BaNa are changed. In BaNa, the Viterbi algorithm is removed and the pitch candidate with the highest confidence score is selected as the estimated pitch for each frame. Similarly, dynamic programming in PEFAC is eliminated and we adopt an earlier version of PEFAC (Gonzalez and Brookes 2011a). The source code for SHRP, HPS, PEFAC, and BaNa are publicly available online (Sun 2002b; Ba 2013; Gonzalez and Brookes 2011b; Ba et al. 2013). The lower and upper limit for pitch are set as 50 and 600 Hz, respectively. The window size is 60 ms and the frame increment step is 10 ms. The rest parameters in the four algorithms are set with the recommended values.

3.4.2 Performance for the Noisy Speeches

3.4.2.1 HPS

Comparing with HPS, the performance of imHPS (achieved by utilizing the proposed iPEEH to HPS) is greatly improved as shown in Fig. 3.4. Here each GPE rate is achieved by averaging over eleven types of noise. In fact, the GPE rate reduction is

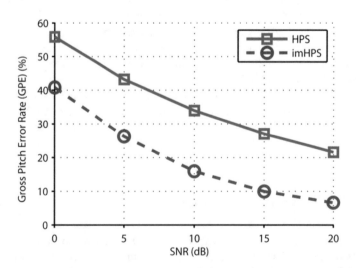

Fig. 3.4 (color online) GPE rate of HPS and imHPS for the LDC database, averaged over all eleven types of noise

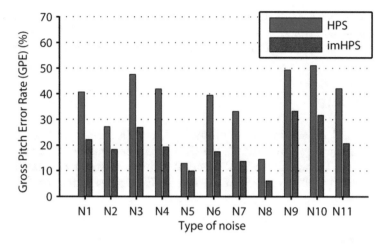

Fig. 3.5 (color online) GPE rate of HPS and imHPS for the LDC database averaged over five SNR levels. The noise types are named as *N1–N11*. Note that the correspondences between the noise types and these short names are shown in Sect. 3.3

over 10% for every SNR level. In addition, performances among different noise types are shown in Fig. 3.5. Obviously, GPE rates of imHPS are all lower than that of HPS for all noise types. Finally, iPEEH is also promising for other datasets, as presented in Fig. 3.6.

The above results show that iPEEH is useful to improve the performance of HPS, which assumes that harmonics in spectrum are precisely linearly distributed and the

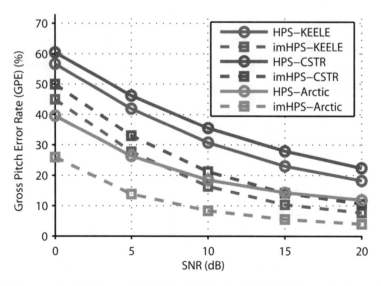

Fig. 3.6 (color online) GPE rate of HPS and imHPS for the KEELE, CSTR, and Arctic databases. Every rate here is averaged over all eleven types of noise

amplitude for each harmonic is distinctive. However, in practice, frequency drift
exists and some harmonics may be missing. The reason why imHPS can achieve
better performance is that iPEEH is effective in supplementing missing harmonics.

3.4.2.2 PEFAC

Similar to HPS, the performance of PEFAC and imPEFAC is compared, as shown in
Fig. 3.7. Comparing with PEFAC, the GPE rates using imPEFAC decrease. For
instance, the GPE rate for the LDC dataset at 20 dB is 16.76% by PEFAC and the
rate declines to 4.34% by imPEFAC. Hence, iPEEH also works for PEFAC.

3.4.2.3 SHRP

As seen from Fig. 3.8, iPEEH is useful to improve SHRP. The key difference
between HPS and SHRP is that SHRP considers the effect of subharmonics. Besides,
the multiplication in HPS is replaced with the addition operation in SHRP. These
two differences enable SHRP less sensitive to the imperfections in a spectrum and
thus SHRP can deal with some unsatisfying spectrums which are likely to cause
failures in HPS. Therefore, the limited improvement for SHRP, in comparison with
HPS, is reasonable.

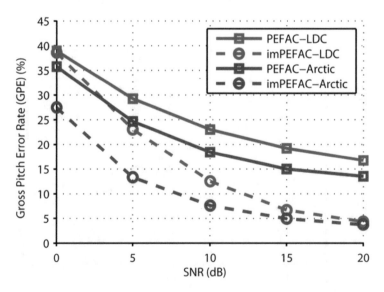

Fig. 3.7 (color online) GPE rate of PEFAC and imPEFAC for the LDC and Arctic databases.
Every rate here is averaged over all eleven types of noise

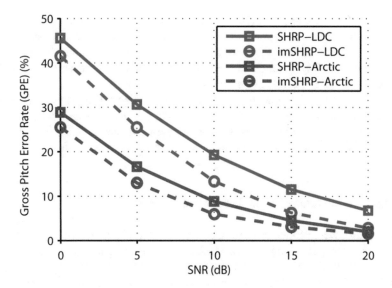

Fig. 3.8 (color online) GPE rate of SHRP and imSHRP for the LDC and Arctic databases. Every rate here is averaged over all eleven types of noise

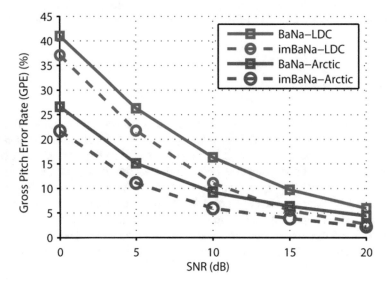

Fig. 3.9 (color online) GPE rate of BaNa and imBaNa for the LDC and Arctic databases. Every rate here is averaged over all eleven types of noise

3.4.2.4 BaNa

Similarly, the comparison is also implemented for BaNa algorithm, as shown in Fig. 3.9. Clearly, imBaNa achieves lower GPE rates than BaNa does for both datasets. However, it is noteworthy that the decline of GPE rate is not as significant as that of HPS. As Yang et al. (2014) have analyzed, BaNa is based on the harmonic ratios and the spectrum amplitude information is ignored once the peaks are selected. Thus, BaNa is in nature more robust to the spectrum amplitude imperfections. Meanwhile, one key function of the iPEEH is to enhance the amplitude of harmonics. Therefore, iPEEH shows limited benefits for BaNa.

From the above experiments, it can be concluded that iPEEH is not only helpful to decrease the estimation errors, but also applicable to multiple frequency-based pitch estimation algorithms. Besides, the comparisons also indicate that iPEEH is effective for noisy speeches of different noise types and SNR levels.

3.4.2.5 Computational Complexity Comparison

Furthermore, we calculate the average processing time per frame (frame length is 60 ms) on a computer using MATLAB R2013a. This computer has an Intel Celeron CPU with 2.60 GHz clock speed and a RAM of 4.00 GB. The results of the running time between the original methods and the corresponding ones after applying iPEEH are calculated, as presented in Table 3.3. Obviously, the running time increases for BaNa and HPS are much larger than that for PEFAC and SHRP. Actually, the differences arise from the FFT length used in each algorithm. As analyzed in Sect. 3.3.4, the processing time for iPEEH is closely related to the FFT length used.

3.4.3 Extension to Music

The proposed method can be further extended to other applications since the harmonics enhancement is valid for other types of periodic signals. For instance, we apply this method to the pitch estimation of music, with the result shown below.

Here, HPS and BaNa (they are both applicable for music) are employed for assessment. For HPS, the upper limit for music pitch is set as 4000 Hz. For BaNa, the source code BaNa-music (Yang et al. 2014; Ba et al. 2013) with post-processing step removed is adopted. As shown in Fig. 3.10, GPE rates indeed decline by using the imHPS and imBaNa-music. On a whole, the average GPE rate decline is 8.72% for HPS and 6.36% for BaNa-music. Thus, the proposed technique is effective even when used for music.

Table 3.3 Elapsed time (in ms) for pitch detection per-frame of speech

Methods	HPS	PEFAC	SHRP	BaNa
Original	6.99	0.98	3.36	49.26
After applying iPEEH	16.04	1.68	3.97	61.26
Difference	9.05	0.70	0.61	12.00

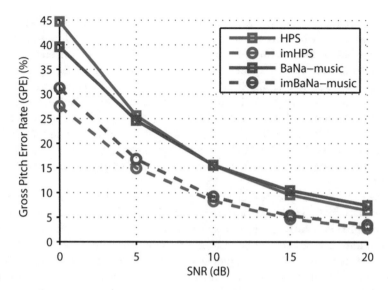

Fig. 3.10 (color online) GPE rate of HPS, imHPS, BaNa, and imBaNa for four pieces of music. Every rate here is averaged over all eleven types of noise

3.4.4 Discussion

As seen from the comparisons, the proposed iPEEH owns strengths in three aspects. (1) It can reduce the pitch detection error. (2) It has extensive applicability. According to the experimental results, iPEEH can be used for different SNR levels, different noise types, and two audio types. Besides, it is one general technique so that it can be embedded into several basic pitch estimators. (3) Novelty. We put forward a creative direction, which is to enhance the harmonics in spectrum first to remove or alleviate poor harmonics structure for harmonics structure improvement before any pitch estimation. One weakness is that it needs extra computation to enhance the harmonics. Besides, iPEEH can deal with the demand when pitch estimation can only be carried out on the single frame.

In addition, there may exist some insights in pitch estimations based on the experiments. Firstly, the main difficulty for many current pitch detection approaches is that speech, especially after contaminated by noise, often shows poor harmonics structure. Secondly, harmonics enhancement before estimation is one feasible solution to improve the pitch detection. And there may be other possible ways for enhancement.

3.5 Summary

In this chapter, we have presented a generalized method iPEEH to improve the performance of many pitch estimation approaches (these in the frequency domain). Starting from investigating the underlying reasons for pitch detection error in existing methods, we found that poor harmonics structure is the main culprit. Based on this discovery, we propose to enhance harmonics in spectrum before adopting any frequency-based pitch estimators. The proposed harmonics enhancement method utilizes the harmonics of a squared speech to supplement the current spectrum and the harmonics structure is improved. Finally, the newly derived spectrum embeds itself into any frequency-based estimation algorithms by replacing the original spectrum. Experimental results show that the proposed iPEEH technique is indeed effective for pitch detection and the GPE rates decline after adopting the iPEEH. Besides, the versatility of the proposed iPEEH is shown since the method is useful for various noise types, multiple noise levels, different original methods, and two audio types.

Based on the analysis and experimental results, we expect that the proposed method is useful for pitch estimation in practice. For the future works, some possible research directions are listed. Firstly, since the iPEEH can be used to deal with every single frame, it is suitable to be utilized for pathological speeches. Note that the traditional methods with global optimization often miss the transient pathological information. Secondly, the proposed iPEEH may offer some inspirations for period estimations of other quasi-periodic signals, such as ECG. Finally, we introduced the idea of harmonics enhancement for pitch estimation. It is meaningful to develop other enhancement approaches and to compare them with the current one.

References

Alonso, J. B., Cabrera, J., Medina, M., & Travieso, C. M. (2015). New approach in quantification of emotional intensity from the speech signal: emotional temperature. *Expert Syst. Appl., 42*(24), 9554-9564.

Ba, H. (2013). Source code for the HPS algorithm. *Available online*: *http://www.ece.rochester.edu/projects/wcng/code/BaNa*.

Ba, H., Yang, N., & Cai, W. (2013). Generated noisy speech data and BaNa source code, WCNG website. *Available online*: *http://www.ece.rochester.edu/projects/wcng/code/BaNa*

Behroozmand, R., Almasganj, F., & Moradi, M. H. (2006). Pathological assessment of vocal fold nodules and polyp using acoustic perturbation and phase space features. In *IEEE International Conference on Acoustics, Speech, and Signal Processing* (pp. II-1056-II-1059).

Bouafif, M., & Lachiri, Z. (2014). Harmonics Enhancement for Determined Blind Sources Separation using Source's Excitation Characteristics. In *International Conference on Control, Engineering & Information Technology Proceedings* (pp. 17-21).

Camacho, A., & Harris, J. G. (2008). A sawtooth waveform inspired pitch estimator for speech and music. *J. Acoust. Soc. Am., 124*(3), 1638-1652.

Chen, S. H., & Wang, J. F. (2002). Noise-robust pitch detection method using wavelet transform with aliasing compensation. *IEE Proc. Vision Image Signal Process., 149*(6), 327-334.

Christensen, M. G., Stoica, P., Jakobsson, A., & Jensen, S. H. (2008). Multi-pitch estimation. *Signal Process., 88*(4), 972-983.

Das, R. (2010). A comparison of multiple classification methods for diagnosis of Parkinson disease. *Expert Syst. Appl., 37*(2), 1568-1572.

De Cheveigne, A., & Kawahara, H. (2002). YIN, a fundamental frequency estimator for speech and music. *J. Acoust. Soc. Am., 111*(4), 1917-1930.

Doweck, Y., Amar, A., & Cohen, I. (2015). Joint Model Order Selection and Parameter Estimation of Chirps with Harmonic Components. *IEEE Trans. Signal Process.*, *63*(7), 1765-1778.

Ercelebi, E. (2003). Second generation wavelet transform-based pitch period estimation and voiced/ unvoiced decision for speech signals. *Appl. Acoust.*, *64*(1), 25-41.

Ghahremani, P., BabaAli, B., Povey, D., Riedhammer, K., Trmal, J., & Khudanpur, S. (2014). A pitch extraction algorithm tuned for automatic speech recognition. In *IEEE International Conference on Acoustics, Speech, and Signal Processing* (pp. 2494-2498).

Gonzalez, S., & Brookes, M. (2011a). A pitch estimation filter robust to high levels of noise (PEFAC). In *19th European Signal Processing Conference* (pp. 451-455).

Gonzalez, S., & Brookes, M. (2011b). Source code for the PEFAC algorithm included in the VOICEBOX toolkit. *Available online*: *http://www.ee.ic.ac.uk/hp/staff/dmb/voicebox/voicebox. html*.

Gonzalez, S., & Brookes, M. (2014). PEFAC - A Pitch Estimation Algorithm Robust to High Levels of Noise. *IEEE/ACM Trans. Audio Speech Lang. Process.*, *22*(2), 518-530.

Hadjitodorov, S., & Mitev, P. (2002). A computer system for acoustic analysis of pathological voices and laryngeal diseases screening. *Med. Eng. Phys.*, *24*(6), 419-429.

Han, K., & Wang, D. (2014). Neural network based pitch tracking in very noisy speech. *IEEE/ACM Trans. Audio Speech Lang. Process.*, *22*(12), 2158-2168.

Huang, F., & Lee, T. (2013). Pitch Estimation in Noisy Speech Using Accumulated Peak Spectrum and Sparse Estimation Technique. *IEEE Trans. Audio Speech Lang. Process.*, *21*(1), 99-109.

Huang, H., & Pan, J. (2006). Speech pitch determination based on Hilbert-Huang transform. *Signal Process.*, *86*(4), 792-803.

Jin, W., Liu, X., Scordilis, M. S., & Han, L. (2010). Speech enhancement using harmonic emphasis and adaptive comb filtering. *IEEE Trans. Audio Speech Lang. Process.*, *18*(2), 356-368.

Kamaruddin, N., Wahab, A., & Quek, C. (2012). Cultural dependency analysis for understanding speech emotion. *Expert Syst. Appl.*, *39*(5), 5115-5133.

Kasuya, H., Ogawa, S., Mashima, K., & Ebihara, S. (1986). Normalized noise energy as an acoustic measure to evaluate pathologic voice. *J. Acoust. Soc. Am.*, *80*(5), 1329-1334.

Kim, S., Eriksson, T., Kang, H. G., & Youn, D. H. (2004). A pitch synchronous feature extraction method for speaker recognition. In *IEEE International Conference on Acoustics, Speech, and Signal Processing* (pp. I-405-I-408).

Kinnunen, T., & Li, H. (2010). An overview of text-independent speaker recognition: From features to supervectors. *Speech comm.*, *52*(1), 12-40.

Krishnamoorthy, P., & Prasanna, S. M. (2010). Two speakers speech separation by LP residual weighting and harmonics enhancement. *Int. J. Speech Technol.*, *13(3)*, 117-139.

Manfredi, C., D'Aniello, M., Bruscaglioni, P., & Ismaelli, A. (2000). A comparative analysis of fundamental frequency estimation methods with application to pathological voices. *Med. Eng. Phys.*, *22*(2), 135-147.

Moran, R. J., Reilly, R. B., De Chazal, P., & Lacy, P. D. (2006). Telephony-based voice pathology assessment using automated speech analysis. *IEEE Trans. Biomed. Eng.*, *53*(3), 468-477.

Naranjo, L., Pérez, C. J., Campos-Roca, Y., & Martín, J. (2016). Addressing voice recording replications for Parkinson's disease detection. *Expert Syst. Appl.*, *46*, 286-292.

Noll, A. M. (1967). Cepstrum pitch determination. *J. Acoust. Soc. Am.*, *41*(2), 293-309.

Plante, F., Meyer, G., & Ainsworth, W. A. (1995). A pitch extraction reference database. In *proceedings of the European Conference on Speech Communication and Technology* (pp.837-840).

Plapous, C., Marro, C., & Scalart, P. (2005). Speech enhancement using harmonic regeneration. In *2005 IEEE International Conference on Acoustics, Speech and Signal Processing* (pp. 157-160).

Qi, Y., & Hillman, R. E. (1997). Temporal and spectral estimations of harmonics-to-noise ratio in human voice signals. *J. Acoust. Soc. Am.*, *102*(1), 537-543.

Rabiner, L. R. (1977). On the use of autocorrelation analysis for pitch detection. *IEEE Trans. Acoust. Speech Signal Process.*, *25*(1), 24-33.

Rao, K. S., Koolagudi, S. G., & Vempada, R. R. (2013). Emotion recognition from speech using global and local prosodic features. *Int. J. Speech Technol.*, *16*(2), 143-160.

Ross, M. J., Shaffer, H. L., Cohen, A., Freudberg, R., & Manley, H. J. (1974). Average magnitude difference function pitch extractor. *IEEE Trans. Acoust. Speech Signal Process.*, *22*(5), 353-362.

Schroeder, M. R. (1968). Period Histogram and Product Spectrum: New Methods for Fundamental-Frequency Measurement. *J. Acoust. Soc. Am.*, *43*(4), 829-834.

Shimamura, T., & Kobayashi, H. (2001). Weighted autocorrelation for pitch extraction of noisy speech. *IEEE Trans. Speech Audio Process.*, *9*(7), 727-730.

Shirota, K., Nakamura, K., Hashimoto, K., Oura, K., Nankaku, Y., & Tokuda, K. (2014). Integration of speaker and pitch adaptive training for HMM-based singing voice synthesis. In *2014 IEEE International Conference on Acoustics, Speech and Signal Processing* (pp. 2559-2563).

Spanias, A. S. (1994). Speech coding: a tutorial review. *Proc. IEEE*, *82*(10), 1541-1582.

Stillwell, J. (2005). *The four pillars of geometry*. Springer Science & Business Media.

Sun, X. (2002a). Pitch determination and voice quality analysis using subharmonic-to-harmonic ratio. In *2002 IEEE International Conference on Acoustics, Speech, and Signal Processing* (pp. I-333-I-336).

Sun, X. (2002b). Source code for the SHRP algorithm. *Available online: http://www.mathworks. com/matlabcentral/fileexchange/1230-pitch-determination-algorithm/content/shrp.m*

Talkin, D. (1995). A robust algorithm for pitch tracking (RAPT). *Speech coding and synthesis*, pp.495-518.

Tao, J., Kang, Y., & Li, A. (2006). Prosody conversion from neutral speech to emotional speech. *IEEE Trans. Audio Speech Lang. Process.*, *14*(4), 1145-1154.

Varga, A., Steeneken, H. J. M., & Jones, D. (1992). The noisex-92 study on the effect of additive noise on automatic speech recognition system. *Reports of NATO Research Study Group (RSG. 10)*.

Wang, Y. B., Li, S. W., & Lee, L. S. (2013). An Experimental Analysis on Integrating Multi-Stream Spectro-Temporal, Cepstral and Pitch Information for Mandarin Speech Recognition. *IEEE Trans. Audio Speech Lang. Process.*, *21*(10), 2006-2014.

Wu, K. B, Zhang, D., Lu, G. M. (2016). iPEEH: Improving pitch estimation by enhancing harmonics. *Expert Systems with Applications. 64*, 317-329.

Wu, J. D., & Lin, B. F. (2009). Speaker identification based on the frame linear predictive coding spectrum technique. *Expert Syst. Appl.*, *36*(4), 8056-8063.

Yang, N., Ba, H., Cai, W., Demirkol, I., & Heinzelman, W. (2014). BaNa: a noise resilient fundamental frequency detection algorithm for speech and music. *IEEE/ACM Trans. Audio, Speech Lang. Process.*, *22*(12), 1833-1848.

Yumoto, E., Gould, W. J., & Baer, T. (1982). Harmonics-to-noise ratio as an index of the degree of hoarseness. *J. Acoust. Soc. Am.*, *71*(6), 1544-1550.

Zavarehei, E., Vaseghi, S., & Yan, Q. (2007). Noisy speech enhancement using harmonic-noise model and codebook-based post-processing. *IEEE Trans. Audio Speech Lang. Process.*, *15*(4), 1194-1203.

Zilca, R. D., Kingsbury, B., Navratil, J., & Ramaswamy, G. N. (2006). Pseudo pitch synchronous analysis of speech with applications to speaker recognition. *IEEE Trans. Audio Speech Lang. Process.*, *14*(2), 467-478.

Chapter 4
Glottal Closure Instants Detection

Abstract Glottal Closure Instants (GCIs) detection is important to many speech applications. However, most existing algorithms cannot achieve computational efficiency and accuracy simultaneously. In this chapter, we present the Glottal closure instants detection based on the Multiresolution Absolute TKEO (GMAT) that can detect GCIs with high accuracy and low computational cost. Considering the nonlinearity in speech production, the Teager–Kaiser Energy Operator (TKEO) is utilized to detect GCIs and an instant with a high absolute TKEO value often indicates a GCI. To enhance robustness, three multiscale pooling techniques, which are max pooling, multiscale product, and mean pooling, are applied to fuse absolute TKEOs of several scales. Finally, GCIs are detected based on the fused results. In the performance evaluation, GMAT is compared with three state-of-the-art methods, MSM (Most Singular Manifold-based approach), ZFR (Zero Frequency Resonator-based method), and SEDREAMS (Speech Event Detection using the Residual Excitation And a Mean-based Signal). On clean speech, experiments show that GMAT can attain higher identification rate and accuracy than MSM. Comparing with ZFR and SEDREAMS, GMAT gives almost the same reliability and higher accuracy. In addition, on noisy speech, GMAT demonstrates the highest robustness for most SNR levels. Additional comparison shows that GMAT is less sensitive to the choice of scale in multiscale processing and it has low computational cost. Finally, pathological speech identification, which is a concrete application of GCIs, is included to show the efficacy of GMAT in practice. Through this chapter, we investigate the potential of TKEO for GCI detection and the proposed algorithm GMAT can detect GCIs with high accuracy and low computational cost. Due to the superiority of GMAT, it will be a promising choice for GCI detection, particularly in real-time scenarios. Hence, this work may contribute to systems relying on GCIs, where both accuracy and computational cost are crucial.

Keywords Glottal closure instants detection · Multiresolution · Teager–Kaiser energy operator (TKEO)

© Springer Nature Singapore Pte Ltd. 2020   75
D. Zhang, K. Wu, *Pathological Voice Analysis*,
https://doi.org/10.1007/978-981-32-9196-6_4

Glottal Closure Instants (GCIs) detection is important to many speech applications. However, most existing algorithms cannot achieve computational efficiency and accuracy simultaneously. In this chapter, we present the Glottal closure instants detection based on the Multiresolution Absolute TKEO (GMAT) that can detect GCIs with high accuracy and low computational cost. Considering the nonlinearity in speech production, the Teager–Kaiser Energy Operator (TKEO) is utilized to detect GCIs and an instant with a high absolute TKEO value often indicates a GCI. To enhance robustness, three multiscale pooling techniques, which are max pooling, multiscale product, and mean pooling, are applied to fuse absolute TKEOs of several scales. Finally, GCIs are detected based on the fused results. In the performance evaluation, GMAT is compared with three state-of-the-art methods, MSM (Most Singular Manifold-based approach), ZFR (Zero Frequency Resonator-based method), and SEDREAMS (Speech Event Detection using the Residual Excitation And a Mean-based Signal). On clean speech, experiments show that GMAT can attain higher identification rate and accuracy than MSM. Comparing with ZFR and SEDREAMS, GMAT gives almost the same reliability and higher accuracy. In addition, on noisy speech, GMAT demonstrates the highest robustness for most SNR levels. Additional comparison shows that GMAT is less sensitive to the choice of scale in multiscale processing and it has low computational cost. Finally, pathological speech identification, which is a concrete application of GCIs, is included to show the efficacy of GMAT in practice. Through this chapter, we investigate the potential of TKEO for GCI detection and the proposed algorithm GMAT can detect GCIs with high accuracy and low computational cost. Due to the superiority of GMAT, it will be a promising choice for GCI detection, particularly in real-time scenarios. Hence, this work may contribute to systems relying on GCIs, where both accuracy and computational cost are crucial.

4.1   Introduction

The detection of glottal closure instant (GCI) is widely needed in speech related applications. A GCI occurs in the production of voiced speech, in which an airflow from the lungs flows through glottis and is modulated by the vibrations of vocal folds. The airflow then reaches vocal tract and finally exits as a sound wave. During this process, vocal folds close and open repeatedly. When air pressure stemming from the lungs increases to a certain degree, the vocal folds are pushed open. The air pressure then decreases after air passes through the glottis, leading to the closure of vocal folds. In each vocal folds vibration, the glottis opens and closes once. GCI refers to the instant of glottal closure in each glottal cycle.

Accurate detection of GCIs is vital for many applications. Voiced speech can be modeled by the source-filter model (Fant 1970), where the source is assumed as a pulse train. In each period of this train, GCI occurs at the instant with the highest amplitude. Hence, GCIs are typically used as the anchor points to model the source of voiced speech (Adiga and Prasanna 2013; Ananthapadmanabha and

Yegnanarayana 1979; Thomas et al. 2009). The significant role of GCIs in source modeling makes it useful for other applications, such as speech coding (Guerchi and Mermelstein 2000) and speech synthesis (Drugman et al. 2009; Moulines and Charpentier 1990). In addition, GCI detection is meaningful in the application of instantaneous pitch tracking (Yegnanarayana and Murty 2009) since detected GCIs can be used to identify individual glottal cycles. Prosodic modification is another application relying on GCIs (Adiga et al. 2014; Rao and Yegnanarayana 2006). GCIs are also useful in pathological speech recognition (Tsanas 2012; Daoudi and Kumar 2015) since detected GCIs can be used to segment voiced speech into successive cycles and the cycle-to-cycle amplitude perturbation is one important dysphonia feature. Moreover, other applications demanding GCI detection include speaker verification (Alku 2011; Murty and Yegnanarayana 2006), speech de-reverberation (Thomas et al. 2007; Gaubitch and Naylor 2007), and causal–anticausal deconvolution (Bozkurt and Dutoit 2003; Drugman et al. 2011).

GCIs can be detected by using electroglottograph (EGG) recordings, which are non-invasive measurements of the vibration of vocal folds during voice production. To obtain the EGG recording, two electrodes are placed on either side of the larynx and the impedance between them is recorded as the EGG signal. Even though GCI detection using EGG is accurate and reliable, the EGG device is often unavailable in practice. In contrast, the device to collect voiced speech (microphone) is more readily available. Hence, researchers have been attracted to study the detection of GCIs when only speech is recorded (no EGG signal). In this chapter, our aim is to develop an automatic GCI detection algorithm for speech.

4.2 Related Works

In this section, many GCI detection algorithms are reviewed and categorized. As to these that are compared with our proposed method in the experiment section, more details are given.

First of all, it is common for numerous GCI detection algorithms to approximate GCIs using various measures in signal-processing field: locations of large values in Linear Prediction Residual (LPR) (Ananthapadmanabha and Yegnanarayana 1979; Drugman and Dutoit 2009; Thomas et al. 2012), lines of maximum amplitudes in wavelet transform (Sturmel et al. 2009; D'Alessandro and Sturmel 2011; Tuan and d'Alessandro 1999), zero crossings after passing the speech to a zero frequency resonator (Murty and Yegnanarayana 2008), and zero crossings of group delay function of LPR (Rao et al. 2007; Naylor et al. 2007; Brookes et al. 2006). Recently, it was claimed that discontinuities estimated under the framework of microcanonical multiscale formalism have relevance to GCIs (Khanagha et al. 2014b). Based on the way to approximate GCI, a majority of GCI detection algorithms can be categorized as follows.

For algorithms based on the LPR, the first step is to compute the LPR from voiced speech. In this stage, speech production is described by the source-filter model and the estimated source is regarded as the LPR. Usually, the filter in this model is simplified as an all-pole type and its coefficients can be estimated by the autoregressive method. With the filter coefficients, the LPR will be obtained by inverse filtering. An ideal LPR signal is an impulse train and the impulse moment within each period coincides with GCI. However, the waveform of LPR for a real speech is much more complicated with many false spikes around the desired peaks (Khanagha et al. 2014b). Thus, multiple approaches are suggested to perform direct or indirect smoothing on the LPR to increase the robustness of GCI estimation. Actually, most algorithms in this category differ only in the way of smoothing. For instance, the Hilbert envelope of LPR was used to find the approximate GCI locations (Rao et al. 2007). The famous DYPSA (Naylor et al. 2007), however, applied the group delay function of LPR to find GCI candidates. In the SEDREAMS algorithm, a mean-based speech was firstly computed to locate a narrow interval for each GCI and then the moment with the highest LPR amplitude inside each narrowed interval was indicated as GCI (Drugman and Dutoit 2009). One variant of LPR is the Integrated Linear Prediction Residual (ILPR). The ILPR signal is obtained by inverse filtering the speech itself (rather than the pre-emphasized speech), whose coefficients are estimated on the pre-emphasized speech. Comparing with the LPR, peaks in the ILPR were demonstrated to be more distinctive (Prathosh et al. 2013). In the YAGA method (Thomas et al. 2012), ILPR was used and a multiscale analysis of ILPR was performed. As suggested by Drugman et al. (2012), smoothing technique is advantageous for LPR-based algorithms. In spite of the direct relationship between GCIs and LPR, LPR is not robust against noise and it often contains peaks of random polarity around CGIs (Murty and Yegnanarayana 2008; Khanagha et al. 2014b). Moreover, LPR-based methods are sensitive to signal polarity (Drugman and Dutoit 2011). More comments on LPR-based algorithms were provided by Murty and Yegnanarayana (2008).

Other GCI detection approaches consider GCIs as discontinuities within each vibration period. Sturmel et al. (2009) adopted wavelet transforms first and then claimed instants with the maximum amplitudes across scales as GCIs. A study in the work of Bouzid and Ellouze (2008) also implemented wavelet transforms at different scales first, but chose to detect GCIs using the product of transformed results. Murty and Yegnanarayana (2008) proposed that GCIs occurred at points with high instantaneous frequencies in a filtered speech. Recently, singularity exponent was introduced into GCI detection (Khanagha et al. 2014b) and points with low singularity exponents were highly unpredictable by their neighbors and thereby corresponded to GCIs in speech. Comparing with the SEDREAMS method (Drugman and Dutoit 2009), the algorithm based on singularity exponent was proved to be more effective for noisy speech and its running time was much lower.

4.2.1   Classical GCI Detection Methods

In the experiments section, three classical state-of-the-art algorithms, namely MSM (Most Singular Manifold-based approach) (Khanagha et al. 2014b), ZFR (Zero Frequency Resonator-based method) (Murty and Yegnanarayana 2008), and the SEDREAMS algorithm (Drugman and Dutoit 2009) are compared with our proposed method. The reasons to add MSM, ZFR, and SEDREAMS methods for comparisons can be found in Sect. 4.4. Here we introduce the three methods briefly.

In MSM, both the criterion to localize GCIs and the way to refine true GCIs from candidates are considered. It is based on a multiscale formalism, which relies on precise estimation of local parameters called Singularity Exponents (SE). The so-called MSM (Most Singular Manifold) is in fact the set of signal samples having the smallest SE values and examples in the paper show that MSM can be adopted for GCI localization. There are three steps in the proposed algorithm:

Step1. *Estimation of the Singularity Exponents*: The singularity exponent of a given signal $s(t)$ can be estimated using the following equation, where r is a scale parameter.

$$\Gamma_r(s(t)) = |2s(t) - s(t-r) - s(t+r)|$$

Step 2. *Multiscale cascading of Singularity Exponents:* By assuming that same singular behavior should be presented across different scale, multiscale fusion was proposed. The final estimation can be expressed as follows, where I is the number of scales and $h_i(t)$ is the log of $\Gamma_{ri}(s(t))$.

$$h(t) = \sum_{i=1}^{I} h_i(t)$$

Step 3. *GCI Detection*: with the computed $h(t)$, GCI can be detected and further refined based on two observations. First, the location of a local minimum of $h(t)$ in each glottal cycle indicates a candidate of GCI. Second, SE values generally decrease suddenly right before each GCI.

Experiments in the paper (Khanagha et al. 2014b) showed that MSM is quite robust against many types of noises and it is computationally efficient. While MSM considers GCIs as discontinuities within each period, the SEDREAM algorithm (Drugman and Dutoit 2009) localizes GCIs based on LPR, which consists of two steps:

Step 1. *Interval determination*: a mean-based signal, which is computed as follows, is used to determine the intervals where GCI was expected to be located. This step is crucial for high identification rate.

$$y(n) = \frac{1}{2N+1} \sum_{m=-N}^{N} \omega(m)s(n+m).$$

Here $w(m)$ is a windowing function and its length is set as 1.75 times the mean pitch period. Note that mean pitch period (and hence pitch estimation) is needed in this approach.

Step 2. *GCI location refinement*: in this step, the precise position of GCIs is assigned by inspecting the LPR within each determined intervals in Step 1. By this refinement, low identification bias can be obtained.

Experiments showed that SEDREAM outperforms the DYPSA algorithm in terms of both accuracy and robustness. Nevertheless, mean pitch period is needed, resulting in more computation and a demand for accurate pitch estimator. As to ZFR, it is based on the assumption that the source of source-filter model in speech production is an impulse train and each impulse moment coincides with GCI for each period. Due to the impulse excitation, the resulted discontinuity is reflected across all the frequencies, including the zero frequency. Therefore, it was proposed in the ZFR algorithm to use a zero frequency filter to detect discontinuity for GCI estimation, in which the "zero frequency" filter was specially chosen to reduce the influence of time-varying vocal tract system. The procedures of ZFR are explained in detail in the following.

Step 1. Compute the difference of the speech signal so that the time-varying low frequency bias in the whole speech can be removed.

Step 2. The differenced speech $x[n]$ is then passed through twice a simply designed zero frequency resonator, as seen below, where $a_1 = -2$ and $a_2 = 1$.

$$y_1[n] = -\sum_{k=1}^{2} a_k y_1[n-k] + x[n]$$

$$y_2[n] = -\sum_{k=1}^{2} a_k y_2[n-k] + y_1[n].$$

Step 3. Subtract the average over 10 ms at each sample to remove the slowly time-varying trend.

After the three above steps, the instants of positive zero crossing in the resulted signal will be assumed as the detected GCIs. Experiments indicated that ZFR gave relatively high identification rates and was robust against several types of noise. In spite of these methods, there exist limitations for accurate and robust GCI detection, as introduced in Sect. 4.2.2.

4.2.2   Limitations

It is worthwhile to mention that many previous methods need pitch information to obtain GCIs. Some rely on pitch to set parameters. In the work of Rao et al. (2007), a Blackman window was employed with its size set as 1.1 times the mean pitch period. Similarly, the pitch knowledge was critical to obtain the mean-based signal in SEDREAMS (Drugman and Dutoit 2009). In the method SE-VQ (Kane and Gobl 2013), estimated pitch was used in the post-processing stage to assist the optimization of GCI detection. Thus, before GCI detection, pitch estimation is demanded, which brings two obvious drawbacks. Firstly, it is often challenging to estimate pitch for expressive and pathological speech. Secondly, extra computation is needed. Thus, it is more desirable to detect GCIs without relying on pitch.

Based on our analysis, the main difficulties in GCI detection are summarized as follows. Firstly, methods based on LPR (ILPR) have to select desired GCIs among peaks with random polarity. Moreover, the time to compute LPR is not negligible. Secondly, pitch estimation is required by many algorithms. However, pitch estimation is challenging under adverse situations and extra calculation is necessary. Thirdly, there are still demands to increase the reliability and accuracy of GCI detection, especially for noisy speech. Finally, the running time of GCI detection is critical for some applications. Hence, we are motivated to propose a GCI detection algorithm with strengths of low computational complexity, high accuracy, and robustness.

Contrary to common assumptions in the source-filter model, complex phenomena exist in speech production (Khanagha 2013b; Teager and Teager 1990; Khanagha et al. 2014a; Teager 1980). With this observation, a nonlinear "energy" operator named TKEO was proposed by Teager (Teager 1980) and Kaiser (Kaiser 1990) to calculate the instantaneous speech "energy." Here it should be pointed that the energy in the notion of TKEO is quite different from the traditional energy, which is the sum of the squares of the signal magnitude. Hereafter, for places with ambiguity, quotation mark is used for "energy" calculated by TKEO. In the proposed method, GCIs are extracted by performing this nonlinear operator TKEO in a multiresolution way. Owing to the excellent properties of TKEO, the proposed method can detect GCIs with high reliability, accuracy, efficiency, and with no requirement of pitch. In addition, the method is robust against noise of many types and levels, less sensitive to parameter change, and suitable for real-time applications. For simplicity, the proposed method is abbreviated as GMAT (GCI detection based on the Multiresolution Absolute TKEO).

The remainder of this chapter is structured as follows. Main methods for GCI detection are reviewed and categorized in Sect. 4.2. The details of the proposed method GMAT are described in Sect. 4.3. In Sect. 4.4, the performance of GMAT is compared with three state-of-the-art methods on four commonly used databases, followed by a brief discussion in Sect. 4.4.2.1. Finally, in Sect. 4.4.2.2, we summarize the chapter and clarify our future works.

4.3   GCI Detection Using TKEO

4.3.1   TKEO and Its Relationship with GCI

Speech production can be modeled by a source-filter model where the vocal tract is assumed as a linear filter system. However, this assumption is not strictly accurate as the vocal tract during speech production is nonlinear in practice (Zhou et al. 2001). Evidence demonstrating nonlinearity in speech was disclosed by H. M. Teager and S. M. Teager (Teager and Teager 1990). Following this work, Kaiser (Kaiser 1990) managed to propose a simple operator to compute the instantaneous speech "energy" with consideration of the nonlinearity. Unlike the conventional energy that considers amplitudes only, the "energy" operator proposed by Kaiser (1990) included the effect of frequencies, showing that speech "energy" depends on both amplitudes and frequencies. This nonlinear "energy" operator (Kaiser 1990) was defined as

$$\Psi[x(t)] = \dot{x}(t)^2 - x(t)\ddot{x}(t), \tag{4.1}$$

where $x(t)$ is a continuous speech and the dot above denotes time derivative. The notation Ψ here represents the "energy" operator TKEO, short for Teager–Kaiser Energy Operator. To use TKEO for discrete time signal, Kaiser derived the discrete form of TKEO:

$$\Psi[x(n)] = x(n)^2 - x(n-1)x(n+1). \tag{4.2}$$

The strengths of TKEO are witnessed by various applications, such as energy separation (Maragos et al. 1993), signal analysis (Ning and Ying 2007; Bahoura and Rouat 2001; Chen et al. 2007; Mitra et al. 1991), speech related recognitions (emotion and speech) (Zhou et al. 2001; Jabloun and Cetin 1999; Kandali et al. 2009), and transient event detection for signal of diverse types (Erdamar et al. 2012; Choi et al. 2006; Pineda-Sanchez et al. 2013; Subasi et al. 2011; Solnik et al. 2010; Nelson et al. 2006). However, only a few works have adopted TKEO to estimate GCIs. Abu-Shikhah and Deriche (1999) proposed estimating pitch by detecting GCIs first where the GCIs were extracted based on the TKEO output. Nevertheless, accuracy of GCI extraction was not the focus of that study. In the work of Patil and Baljekar (2011), it was demonstrated with an example that peaks in the VTEO (Variable length Teager Energy Operator) were in close proximity to the locations of the corresponding GCIs. Another study (Patil and Viswanath 2011) used TKEO to improve GCI estimation for voiced speech and to alleviate any wrong detection in unvoiced regions as well, aiming to achieve good overall performance for both voiced and unvoiced regions. If only voiced regions were considered, this algorithm yielded much lower identification rate comparing with the ZFR method (Murty and Yegnanarayana 2008). Hence, the potential of operator TKEO for GCI detection needs further investigation.

In this book, we exploit TKEO to estimate GCIs and our motivations are based on the following considerations. First, TKEO reflects the instantaneous "energy" and only three samples are needed to calculate the "energy" for each instant. This outstanding resolution makes it suitable to detect discontinuities. Secondly, high efficiency can be achieved since TKEO calculation is extremely simple. This merit marks its distinct significance in real-time applications. Thirdly, TKEO can be used for non-stationary signals (Banerjee and Chakrabarti 2015). Hence, when TKEO is applied, there is no need to split a speech into overlapping frames like LPR (Mitra et al. 2012). Fourthly, TKEO can be regarded as a high-pass filter. Studies show that TKEO was able to enhance the high frequency portions of a given signal (Subasi et al. 2011; Mukhopadhyay and Ray 1998) and local discontinuities could be captured. Finally, combining multiresolution techniques with TKEO may further boost the performance. Research on the application of action potential detection indicates that multiresolution TKEO provides considerable improvements (Choi et al. 2006; Choi and Kim 2002). With these properties, it is reasonable to apply TKEO to detect GCIs.

4.3.2 Absolute TKEO with Scale Parameter k

Literature shows that operator TKEO can be used to detect discontinuities (Drira et al. 2014; Pantazis et al. 2005; Ulriksen and Damkilde 2016). In voiced speech, discontinuities often occur at the instants of glottal closure. Therefore, it is reasonable to utilize TKEO for GCI detection.

In the definition of discrete TKEO, it takes three samples for calculation. If one point $x(n)$ is a discontinuity, then amplitudes of its backward point $x(n-1)$ and forward point $x(n+1)$ often differ greatly from $x(n)$, resulting in a large absolute TKEO output. On the contrary, the amplitude differences between non-discontinuity points and their consecutive points are rather small, leading to low absolute TKEO results. The absolute TKEO is defined as:

$$|\Psi[x(n)]| = \left|x(n)^2 - x(n-1)x(n+1)\right|. \tag{4.3}$$

Note that the absolute operation is added. For briefness, the absolute TKEO defined above is denoted as *aTKEO* thereafter. Obviously, the operator *aTKEO* can measure local changes and thus provides a way to identify discontinuities.

Intuitively, if we apply the operator *aTKEO* to a voiced speech, then points with large outputs may correspond to GCIs. However, since only three samples are adopted, the output of *aTKEO* is highly sensitive, especially for noisy speech. To handle the sensitivity of TKEO, Choi and Kim (2002) proposed adding a resolution parameter k to the traditional TKEO, denoted as k-TEO. The definition of k-TEO is:

$$\Theta_k\{x(n)\} = x(n)^2 - x(n-k)x(n+k). \tag{4.4}$$

In this equation, parameter k is a positive integer, measuring the time distance between $x(n-k)$ (or $x(n+k)$) and $x(n)$. When k is equal to 1, k-TEO is reduced to the traditional TKEO. The capacity of operator k-TEO in capturing "energy" of speech was investigated with the name Variable Length Teager Energy Operator (VTEO) (Tomar and Patil 2008). Following this idea, we define the scale parameter for *aTKEO*:

$$|\Psi_k[x(n)]| = |x(n)^2 - x(n-k)x(n+k)|. \tag{4.5}$$

A larger k indicates a larger scale so that the involved samples in Eq. (4.5) are further away from each other and the relevance between them decreases. Thereafter, the absolute TKEO with scale parameter k is assigned with a notion $\Omega(k)$.

4.3.3 Multiresolution Combination

To enhance robustness of GCI detection, the idea of multiresolution combination has been frequently used in previous GCI detection, especially in methods based on wavelet transform (Thomas et al. 2012; Sturmel et al. 2009; D'Alessandro and Sturmel 2011; Tuan and d'Alessandro 1999). Applying multiresolution combination is beneficial in two regards. Firstly, a multiscale method covers more local samples and thus it can enhance robustness. Secondly, features of transient events are often displayed across multiple scales. Therefore, we perform a multiresolution *aTKEO* to improve GCI detection.

In this section, we combine multiple absolute TKEO $\Omega(k)$ with scale parameter k varying from 1 to M. In general, there are three common pooling approaches. One is the max pooling, which is to use the maximum filter in a pointwise way (Choi et al. 2006; Choi and Kim 2002). The second way to combine multiresolution results is the multiscale product. For instance, the GCI detection method proposed by Thomas et al. (2012) was based on the multiscale product of stationary wavelet transform results. Usually, computing multiscale product is realized according to the logarithmic summation rule. The last fusing approach is average pooling, in which the fused result is equal to the pointwise average. With the three pooling techniques, fused outcomes are formulated, respectively:

$$p_1(n) = \max\left(|\Psi_1[x(n)]|, \frac{1}{2}|\Psi_2[x(n)]|, \ldots, \frac{1}{M}|\Psi_M[x(n)]|\right); \tag{4.6}$$

$$p_2(n) = \sum_{k=1}^{M} \log\left(|\Psi_k[x(n)]|/k\right); \tag{4.7}$$

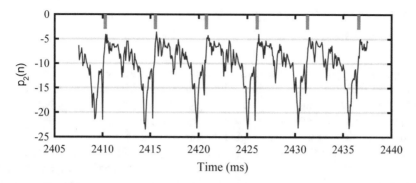

Fig. 4.1 (color online) The signal $p_2(n)$ varies with time. Time-aligned GCIs ground truths are marked with green vertical lines

$$p_3(n) = \sum_{k=1}^{M} \frac{1}{k} |\Psi_k[x(n)]|. \tag{4.8}$$

Note that the multiscale product is realized by logarithmic summation as in Eq. (4.7) (Here M is the number of scales used in fusion. Detailed analysis of this parameter is provided in Sect. 4.4.2.1). Additionally, a weight $1/k$ is given to $\Omega(k)$ in the multiscale combination. The weighting scheme is reasonable since adjacent samples contribute more in computing local changes for a discontinuity and distant samples are less related. Instants in $p_2(j)$ with amplitudes of negative infinite are set with the average of $p_2(n)$. With the three pooling techniques in Eqs. (4.6), (4.7) and (4.8), the resulting GCI detection algorithms are named as GMAT$_{max}$, GMAT$_{prod}$, and GMAT$_{mean}$, respectively. Their performances are compared experimentally in Sect. 4.4. In this section, we take the multiscale product method GMAT$_{prod}$ as an example to describe the remaining steps.

According to our preceding analysis, the *aTKEO* output for a discontinuity should be distinct. Besides, geometric features of discontinuities are often exhibited across multiple scales. Thus, the multiscale pooling output $p_2(n)$ should have large amplitudes for points neighboring GCIs. For demonstration, one example is presented in Fig. 4.1. Here, the speech segment is from the SLT database (Kominek and Black 2004) and the scale number parameter M is set to nine. Green vertical lines in Fig. 4.1 represent the locations of GCI ground truths derived from the matched EEG signal. The way to derive GCIs from EEG is given in detail in Sect. 4.4. From this figure, it is evident that there are sudden positive peaks around GCIs in signal $p_2(n)$. This observation is in consistence with our analysis.

4.3.4 GMAT: GCI Detection Based on Multiresolution Absolute TKEO

In Fig. 4.1, it is observed that GCI points in $p_2(n)$ always have larger amplitudes, compared with their local samples within one period. However, when comparing with points outside the pitch period, the $p_2(n)$ amplitudes of GCI points are not always the highest, due to the fluctuation of the $p_2(n)$ envelope. Hence, GCIs cannot be extracted directly by using a global threshold on signal $p_2(n)$.

There are predominantly two approaches to coping with the current difficulties. One is to estimate pitch period first and then to limit the peak detection within a single period. For instance, SEDREAMS method employed the average pitch to design a low-pass filter and the filtered speech was utilized to localize a narrow interval in each period that includes GCI (Drugman and Dutoit 2009). Then point with the highest LPR in each interval was regarded as GCI. However, pitch estimation brings in extra computation and the resulting overall efficiency will be low. On the other hand, the alternative method, which is to perform a simple but effective post-processing (Khanagha et al. 2014b), is much more efficient and pitch estimation is unnecessary. In essence, the solution was to define a high-pass filter to reduce envelope fluctuation and the filtered signal could measure the average deviation in local region. As shown in Fig. 4.1, sudden amplitude rises of $p_2(n)$ right before GCIs are evident. Hence, one filter is devised to detect the sudden rise:

$$q(n) = \frac{1}{T_l} \left(\sum_{j=n}^{n+T_l} p_2(j) - \sum_{j=n-T_l}^{n-1} p_2(j) \right). \tag{4.9}$$

This filter computes the average change of $p_2(n)$ after and before the sudden rises in each period. Based on our analysis, signal $q(n)$ should show large peaks around GCIs. The parameter T_l here represents the window length to compute the average change. In this book, this parameter is assigned to the integer nearest to $2.5f_s/1000$ (f_s is the sampling rate of speech). A detailed analysis of this parameter is presented in Sect. 4.4.2.1. Applying Eq. (4.9) to $p_2(n)$ in Fig. 4.1, the calculated $q(n)$ is shown in Fig. 4.2. Note that the waveform of $q(n)$ in Fig. 4.2 has been scaled to display. Evidently, high peaks in $q(n)$ are located near the peaks in $p_2(n)$ and thereby near the ground truth GCIs.

Comparing with $p_2(n)$, signal $q(n)$ has two highlights. On one hand, it is more robust to noise. Since $q(n)$ represents the average deviation over samples in a window of T_l, a hidden smoothing effect is included, which makes the signal $q(n)$ more robust to additive noise. On the other hand, $q(n)$ is less affected by the envelope fluctuation owning to the effect of the high-pass filter. In our method GMAT, signal $q(n)$ is combined with $p_2(n)$ to attain desirable outcomes.

The implementation details of GMAT are described as follows. Firstly, calculate $p_2(n)$ and $q(n)$ according to Eqs. (4.7) and (4.9), respectively. Secondly, positive portions of $q(n)$ are segmented out by its zero crossings. Thirdly, within each

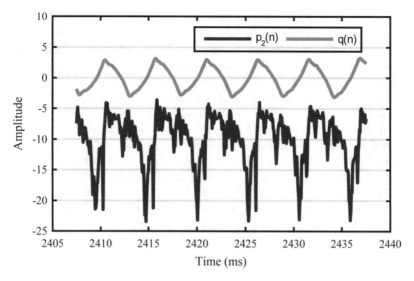

Fig. 4.2 (color online) The signal $q(n)$ is shown with green color. The signal $p_2(n)$ in Fig. 4.1 is added for comparison. Notice that $q(n)$ has been scaled for better display

positive portion, the instant with the highest $q(n)$ is detected, denoted as n_1. Fourthly, in the same positive portion, instants with the first three highest $p_2(n)$ are identified and the one closest to n_1 is represented as n_2. Finally, instant n_3, which is the average of n_1 and n_2, is taken as the estimated GCI within this period.

The rationale behind step 2–5 is explained. In step 2, each segmented positive portion is used to localize a narrow interval that includes GCI. The followed steps are to refine GCI location in this interval. Intuitively, it seems that the instant with the highest $p_2(n)$ in each segmented positive region, denoted as n_0, should correspond to an estimation of GCI. Nevertheless, it is noteworthy that each segmented positive portion gives a rather fuzzy region where a GCI could happen. In this region, there may be many false spikes in signal $p_2(n)$, especially when the speech is corrupted with noise. Hence, analyzing peaks in signal $p_2(n)$ only is not sufficient to detect GCI accurately. In fact, step 3, 4, and 5 are introduced such that the refinement of GCI detection can be more robust and accurate. Besides the instant with high amplitude, the sudden rise in signal $p_2(n)$ also indicates a GCI and the rise is shown as a peak in each positive portion of signal $q(n)$. As illustrated in Fig. 4.2, signal $q(n)$ is much more robust than $p_2(n)$ and its single peak in each segmented interval is often located near the ground truth GCI. Hence, the instant with the highest $q(n)$ in each interval, denoted as n_1, is detected in step 3. The meaning of detecting the instant n_1 is twofold. First, it is located near the ground truth GCI, offering another GCI estimation. Second, it helps to guide the peak picking on signal $p_2(n)$ since the true GCI should occur in the neighborhood of n_1. In the followed fourth step, three instants in $p_2(n)$ are first detected and then instant n_1 is used to guide picking the nearest one n_2. Three instants are used to handle the possible false spikes in $p_2(n)$. Both n_1 and n_2 give a GCI estimation and their ability in refining GCI locations varies with our pooling techniques. For instance, when product pooling is used, as in Eq. (4.7), instant n_2 is more precise at predicting GCI. In contrast, in case of average pooling, the preciseness of n_2 is alleviated due to the averaging operation and instant n_1 can predict GCI more accurately. Since the GCI refining scheme remains the same for $GMAT_{max}$, $GMAT_{prod}$, and $GMAT_{mean}$, the average of n_1 and n_2 is taken in step 5 to enhance robustness. For more evidences, instants n_0, n_1, and n_2 are taken as GCI estimations to compare with n_3 experimentally in Sect. 4.4.

Obviously, the proposed GMAT algorithm needs no pitch information to detect GCIs and thus pitch estimation is unnecessary. Besides, comparing with methods based on LPR, GMAT is performed directly speech. Note that LPR is calculated frame by frame and each frame of LPR needs auto-regression coefficient estimation and inverse filtering. Therefore, GMAT should be of comparatively high efficiency. Before the end of this section, it is worthwhile to notice that the analysis and operations of $p_2(n)$ in Sect. 4.3.3 are applicable to $p_1(n)$ and $p_3(n)$.

4.4 Experimental Results

In this section, we compare the proposed method GMAT against three state-of-the-art algorithms: the Most Singular Manifold-based approach (MSM) presented by Khanagha et al. (2014b), the Zero Frequency Resonator-based method (ZFR) proposed by Murty and Yegnanarayana (2008), and the famous SEDREAMS algorithm (Drugman and Dutoit 2009). With regard to GMAT, $GMAT_{max}$, $GMAT_{prod}$, and $GMAT_{mean}$ are all considered. They differ only in the way of multiresolution pooling, as described in Sect. 4.3.2.

In this following, we first evaluate the GCI detection performances for both clean and noisy speech before the scheme to refine GCI location for GMAT is analyzed. In Sect. 4.4.2.1, the sensitivity of scale parameter M and window length parameter T_l is tested, followed by the assessment of running time. Finally, one practical application of GCI detection, which is to assist extracting extraction in pathological speech recognition task, is included to assess the ability of GCI detection methods in practical task. Through comparisons, it is demonstrated that the GMAT algorithm has certain advantages over MSM, ZFR, and SEDREAMS.

More detailed description of the experimental settings and results can be found in the work of (Wu et al. 2017).

4.4.1 Basic Experimental Settings

The performance of GCI detection algorithm is assessed by comparing GCIs extracted from speech with the ground truth GCIs derived from EGG signals. In this section, four freely available online databases (Kominek and Black 2004) are applied. One is the KED, while the other three are taken from the CMU ARCTIC

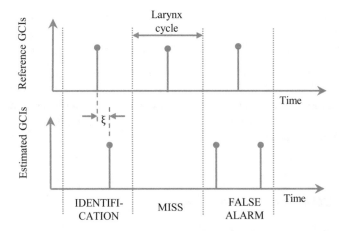

Fig. 4.3 (color online) Characterization of GCIs extraction with three possible outcomes (Thomas et al. 2007): identification, miss, and false alarm. The notion ξ denotes timing error

database. Before experiments, all speech and EGG recordings are resampled at 16 kHz and speech are time-aligned with the corresponding EGG recordings to remove the larynx-to-microphone delay.

The evaluations are also performed on noisy speech, which is generated by mixing clean speech with pure noise of different types. Clean speech is taken from the four introduced databases. For the pure noise, 12 types of noise taken from the NOISEX-92 (Varga et al. 1992) are applied: babble noise (*N1*), destroyer engine room noise (*N2*), destroyer operations room noise (*N3*), F-16 cockpit noise (*N4*), factory floor noise (*N5*), high frequency radio channel noise (*N6*), military vehicle noise (*N7*), tank noise (*N8*), machine gun noise (*N9*), pink noise (*N10*), vehicle interior noise (*N11*), and white noise (*N12*). SNRs (signal-to-noise ratio) for the noisy speech are in 11 levels from −20 to 30 dB.

Generally, GCI ground truths derived from EGG signals occur at the instant with the highest differentiated EGG (dEGG). In this section, we used the online available code (Khanagha 2013a) to detect GCI ground truths from dEGG. The evaluation methodology in Thomas et al. (2012) is used to measure the performance of GCI detection algorithm objectively. As depicted in Fig. 4.3, each larynx cycle is defined by the ground truth GCIs. Assuming that the kth reference GCI is located at m_k, then the kth larynx cycle should include samples in the range of $((m_{k-1} + m_k)/2, (m_k + m_{k+1})/2)$. Comparing the location of the detected GCI with that of the reference GCI in each defined larynx cycle, two classes of measurements can be defined. The measurements in the first class describe the reliability of GCI detection:

- Identification Rate (IDR): the percentage of larynx cycles with one detected GCI.
- Miss Rate (MR): the percentage of larynx cycles with no detected GCI.
- False Alarm Rate (FAR): the percentage of larynx cycles with more than one detected GCI.

In addition to reliability, another concern is accuracy. For each larynx cycle counted in the calculation of IDR, the timing error between the reference GCI and the detected GCI is denoted as ξ. There are then two criteria for measuring accuracy:

- Identification Accuracy (IDA): the standard deviation of timing error ξ. A lower IDA is desired.
- Identification Bias (IDB): the mean of the absolute timing error. Note that the mean is computed over the absolute timing error to avoid error cancellation. A lower IDB is preferred.

4.4.2 Performance Comparison

4.4.2.1 GCI Detection for Clean Speech

Table 4.1 presents the performance on clean speech. First, we compare GMAT against the ZFR algorithm: ZFR generally gives higher IDRs than GMAT, while ZFR leads to highest identification biases. Comparing with MSM, we find that the IDRs of $GMAT_{max}$, $GMAT_{prod}$, and $GMAT_{mean}$ surpass that of MSM on all four databases. With regard to accuracy, MSM always reaches higher IDA than GMAT on all four databases. In the comparison with SEDREAMS, SEDREAMS achieves higher IDRs than GMAT on all four databases except on JMK database. As to the accuracy metrics, GMAT variants have lower IDAs and IDBs than SEDREAM in an average sense.

Moreover, we also compare the three GMAT based approaches with each other. For reliability, the IDR of $GMAT_{mean}$ is slightly higher than that of $GMAT_{prod}$, whereas $GMAT_{max}$ gives the lowest. $GMAT_{max}$ provides the lowest IDA and IDB on average. Meanwhile, $GMAT_{prod}$ and $GMAT_{mean}$ have comparable accuracy performance.

In summary, the ZFR and SEDREAMS algorithms outperform GMAT in terms of reliability, whereas GMAT is superior to MSM. As to accuracy, GMAT reaches the lowest IDA and IDB among all methods in comparison. Specially, SEDREAMS generally leads to the highest identification rate and ZFR always results in the largest identification bias. Furthermore, three pooling techniques for GMAT show similar performances, with $GMAT_{mean}$ having a slim advantage regarding IDR and $GMAT_{max}$ gaining a slightly higher accuracy.

4.4.2.2 GCI Detection for Noisy Speech

In this part, we use IDR to measure reliability and IDB to indicate accuracy. Notice that each IDR and IDB shown is achieved by averaging over 4 databases and 12 noise types. The performances under different SNR levels are shown in Figs. 4.4 and 4.5. Figures 4.6 and 4.7 are added to highlight the performance

Table 4.1 Performance comparisons of GCI detection algorithms on clean speeches

Database	Method	IDR (%)	FAR (%)	MR (%)	IDA (ms)	IDB (ms)
KED	MSM	97.19	1.66	1.15	0.45	0.30
	ZTFR	98.45	1.25	0.30	0.64	2.38
	SEDREAMS	**99.51**	**0.35**	**0.15**	0.51	0.41
	GMA_{max}	97.88	1.57	0.54	**0.30**	**0.19**
	$GMAT_{prod}$	97.77	1.74	0.49	0.38	0.24
	$GMAT_{mean}$	97.95	1.46	0.60	0.42	0.24
BDL	MSM	93.99	2.72	3.29	0.61	0.29
	ZFR	96.21	1.79	**2.00**	**0.40**	0.75
	SEDREAMS	**97.17**	**0.78**	2.05	0.51	**0.22**
	$GMAT_{max}$	95.41	1.90	2.70	0.52	0.32
	$GMAT_{prod}$	96.15	1.18	2.67	0.52	0.29
	$GMAT_{mean}$	96.07	1.18	2.75	0.54	0.32
JMK	MSM	94.04	3.46	2.50	0.65	0.32
	ZFR	**97.68**	0.25	2.07	0.63	1.57
	SEDREAMS	97.64	**0.21**	2.15	0.62	0.40
	$GMAT_{max}$	95.33	2.50	2.17	**0.56**	0.33
	$GMAT_{prod}$	95.67	2.36	**1.97**	**0.56**	0.35
	$GMAT_{mean}$	95.86	2.01	2.12	0.57	**0.31**
SLT	MSM	96.22	1.15	2.62	0.38	**0.23**
	ZFR	98.75	0.94	0.31	**0.23**	0.63
	SEDREAMS	**98.79**	1.14	**0.07**	0.31	0.24
	$GMAT_{max}$	97.36	0.96	1.68	0.36	0.27
	$GMAT_{prod}$	97.47	1.04	1.49	0.34	0.25
	$GMAT_{mean}$	97.30	**0.93**	1.76	0.34	**0.23**
Overall	MSM	95.36	2.25	2.39	0.52	0.29
	ZFR	97.77	1.06	1.17	0.48	1.33
	SEDREAMS	**98.28**	**0.62**	**1.10**	0.49	0.32
	$GMAT_{max}$	96.49	1.73	1.77	**0.44**	**0.28**
	$GMAT_{prod}$	96.77	1.58	1.65	0.45	**0.28**
	$GMAT_{mean}$	96.80	1.40	1.81	0.47	**0.28**

Bold values indicate better results

differences when SNR ranges from 0 to 30 dB. In summary, comparing with ZFR, the GMAT based algorithms $GMAT_{prod}$ and $GMAT_{mean}$ have better robustness against additive noise, achieving higher reliability and accuracy for most SNR levels.

In comparison with MSM, $GMAT_{mean}$ and $GMAT_{prod}$ achieve higher IDRs for all 11 SNR levels, while $GMAT_{max}$ obtains higher IDRs only when SNR is over 0 dB. As for accuracy, it is observed in Figs. 4.5 and 4.7 that MSM tends to give higher IDBs than GMAT at positive SNR levels. It can be concluded that the three GMAT variants are more advantageous than MSM in terms of both reliability and accuracy, especially when the SNR is over 0 dB.

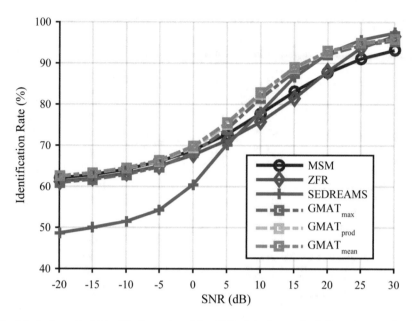

Fig. 4.4 (color online) Identification rates of five GCIs detection methods for noisy speech with different noise levels. Note that each rate here is achieved by averaging over 12 types of noise and 4 databases

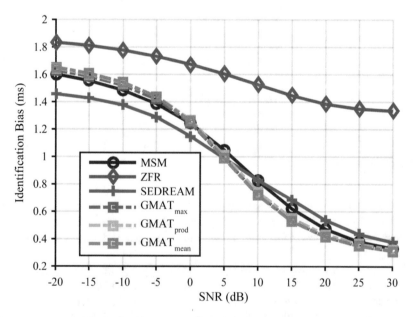

Fig. 4.5 (color online) Identification biases of five GCI detection methods for noisy speech with different noise levels. Note that each bias here is achieved by averaging over 12 types of noise and 4 databases

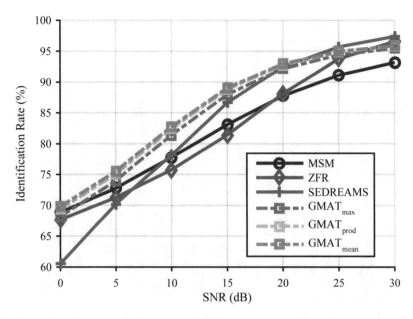

Fig. 4.6 (color online) Identification rates of five GCIs detection methods for noisy speech with SNR ranging from 0 to 30 dB. Note that each rate here is achieved by averaging over 12 types of noise and 4 databases

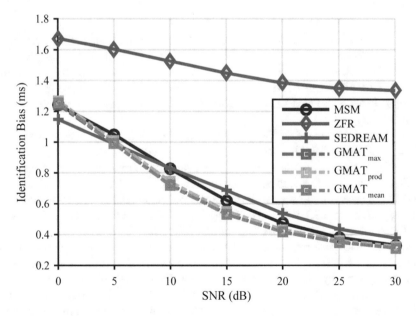

Fig. 4.7 (color online) Identification biases of five GCI detection methods for noisy speech with SNR ranging from 0 to 30 dB. Note that each bias here is achieved by averaging over 12 types of noise and 4 databases

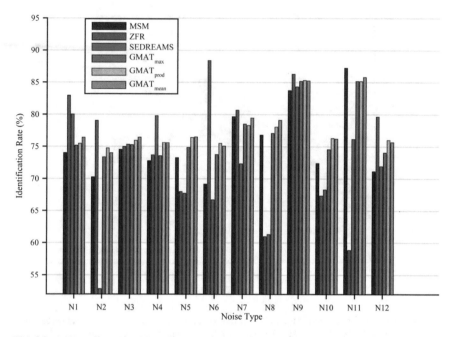

Fig. 4.8 (color online) Identification rates of five GCI estimation methods for noisy speech with different noise types. Note that each rate here is calculated by averaging over 11 SNR levels and 4 databases

In addition, as illustrated in Fig. 4.4, GMAT variants offer higher IDRs than SEDREAMS up to 20 dB of SNR. As to accuracy, GMAT based algorithms give lower IDBs when SNR is over 5 dB and they reach slightly higher averaged IDBs than SEDREAMS. Since IDB is defined only for larynx cycles counted in IDR, it is reasonable to choose GMAT over SEDREAMS for noisy speech, especially in case of low SNR.

To compare among $GMAT_{max}$, $GMAT_{prod}$, and $GMAT_{mean}$, Figs. 4.4 and 4.6 show that the reliability performances are ranked in a descending order as $GMAT_{mean}$, $GMAT_{prod}$, and $GMAT_{max}$ for every considered SNR level. According to Figs. 4.5 and 4.7, they can be ranked (descending) as $GMAT_{prod}$, $GMAT_{mean}$, and $GMAT_{max}$ based on the average IDB. As mentioned, the indicator IDB is meaningful only after the IDR is also taken into consideration. Overall, $GMAT_{mean}$ outperforms $GMAT_{prod}$ and $GMAT_{max}$ for noisy speech.

Furthermore, performance comparisons for various noise types are presented in Figs. 4.8 and 4.9. First, ZFR and GMAT both have superior IDRs in 4 noise types. Regarding accuracy, ZFR still gives the highest IDBs for all noise types, suggesting a lower accuracy. Comparing with MSM, GMAT based algorithms have higher IDRs for most noise types, except for *N7* and *N11*. In the comparison with SEDREAMS, GMAT outperforms GMAT for most types, except for noise type *N1* and *N4* in terms of reliability. As for the IDB metric, it is observed that SEDREAMS gives lower IDBs for seven noise types, while GMAT is more

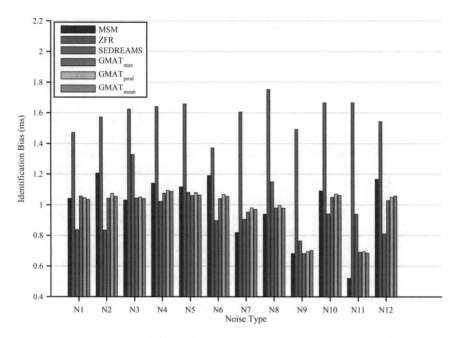

Fig. 4.9 (color online) Identification biases of five GCI estimation methods for noisy speech with different noise types. Note that each bias here is obtained by averaging over 11 SNR levels and 4 databases

beneficial for the other five types. Hence, GMAT has advantages over SEDREAMS for most noise types. When performing comparisons among $GMAT_{max}$, $GMAT_{prod}$, and $GMAT_{mean}$, $GMAT_{mean}$ performs better for more noise types.

Our evaluations on noisy speech lead to meaningful conclusions. Firstly, comparing with ZFR, GMAT based methods often lead to higher IDRs for most SNR levels. In terms of accuracy, GMAT is much more advantageous than ZFR, either for different SNR levels or for noise types. However, ZFR displays high robustness against four noise types (babble noise, destroyer engine room noise, high frequency radio channel noise, and white noise). Secondly, GMAT based algorithms demonstrate better performances in terms of both reliability and accuracy in comparison with MSM when the SNR is over 0 dB. In case of negative SNRs, MSM is more accurate than GMAT, whereas GMAT is more reliable. Thirdly, GMAT reaches distinctly higher identification rates than SEDREAMS on speech of low SNRs and ten noise types. Finally, $GMAT_{max}$, $GMAT_{prod}$, and $GMAT_{mean}$ have similar performances. In detail, $GMAT_{max}$ still has the lowest GCI detection bias and $GMAT_{mean}$ reaches the highest IDR as in the scenario of clean speech. On the negative side, however, we notice that the MSM algorithm can cope with noise type N7 and N11 better than GMAT, which is explained in detail in Sect. 4.4.2.1.

4.4.2.3 Analysis of GCI Refinement Scheme

Section 4.3.4 introduces the scheme to refine GCI locations in the proposed GMAT. Here, an experiment is added to demonstrate the validity of our refinement solution.

To detect GCI, each positive portion of signal $q(n)$ is firstly segmented and it is regarded as the narrow interval where a GCI is expected to occur. In fact, the average interval lengths (on four clean datasets) for three multiresolution pooling methods (max, product, and mean) are 46.8, 52.1, and 53.1 samples, respectively. To find GCI among the samples, location refinement is needed. In Sect. 4.3.4, four locations, denoted as n_0, n_1, n_2, and n_3, are presented. Here we compare their preciseness in refining GCI location.

Metrics IDR and IDB are employed in the comparison and the results are shown in Table 4.2. It can be seen that using n_0 to refine GCI location gives the highest bias, indicating that relying on peaks in $p_2(n)$ alone is not enough to detect GCI accurately. Further, using n_1 as the GCI has higher accuracy for maxing pooling and mean pooling. Meanwhile, applying n_2 to refine GCI is more advantageous for $GMAT_{prod}$. Hence, the average of n_1 and n_2 is taken as the final GCI in GMAT to achieve better performance.

4.4.2.4 Comparison of Running Time

Running time is an important consideration for GCI detection algorithms, especially in real-time applications. In this part, we compare the running time of ZFR, MSM, SEDREAMS, and GMAT.

Table 4.2 Comparisons for different schemes of GCI location refinement

Pooling	Refining method	IDR (%)	IDB (ms)
$GMAT_{max}$	n_0	96.25	0.496
	n_1	**96.49**	0.283
	n_2	**96.49**	0.286
	$n_3 = (n_1 + n_2)/2$	**96.49**	**0.276**
$GMAT_{prod}$	n_0	96.61	0.499
	n_1	96.45	0.470
	n_2	96.74	**0.267**
	$n_3 = (n_1 + n_2)/2$	**96.77**	0.283
$GMAT_{mean}$	n_0	96.59	0.508
	n_1	96.78	0.319
	n_2	**96.80**	0.339
	$n_3 = (n_1 + n_2)/2$	**96.80**	**0.278**
Overall	n_0	96.48	0.501
	n_1	96.57	0.357
	n_2	96.68	0.297
	$n_3 = (n_1 + n_2)/2$	**96.69**	**0.279**

Bold values indicate better results

Table 4.3 Normalized running time (NPT) comparisons

Methods	MSM	ZFR	SEDREAMS	$GMAT_{max}$	$GMAT_{prod}$	$GMAT_{mean}$
NPT(ms)	16.25	**2.56**	58.14	11.02	15.77	10.79

Bold values indicate better results

The running time consumed for each speech is normalized by the speech duration, which represents the time consumed to detect GCI for speech with a length of one second. In this experiment, the computer has an Intel Core i3 CPU with 2.40 GHz clock speed and 4.00 GB of RAM. All algorithms are implemented using MATLAB R2015a. The results in Table 4.3 are normalized running times (NRT) averaged over four clean databases. Note that the NRT of SEDREAMS here does not include the time of estimating the average pitch.

As in Table 4.3, the NRT of MSM is longer than all three GMAT variants. ZFR is the fastest. SEDREAMS, however, is much more time-consuming comparing with other methods. Four conclusions are then drawn. First, ZFR is recommended when running time is extremely crucial. Second, in comparison with MSM, GMAT based algorithms have lower or equal computational costs. Besides, NRT of GMAT can be reduced at the cost of a slight performance reduction since GMAT is not as sensitive to scale number as MSM. Third, $GMAT_{prod}$ is less efficient than $GMAT_{max}$ and $GMAT_{mean}$, which may be caused by the logarithmic operation in $GMAT_{prod}$. Fourth, ZFR, MSM, and GMAT all take less than 17 ms to detect GCIs for a speech of 1 s, making them feasible in real-time applications. Note that NRT of SEDREAMS is nearly 1 s and the time to estimate pitch should also be included.

4.4.3   GCIs Detection in Pathological Speech Identification

Voice is a biomedical signal that can be used to detect disease symptoms. Tsanas (2012) used voice for automatic Parkinson's disease diagnosis and monitoring, in which some dysphonia features rely on GCI detection. In this part, the performance of GMAT in a practical application, which is speech based pathology recognition, is explored.

Our goal is to discriminate patients with Parkinson's disease (PWP) from healthy subjects by voice analysis. For this purpose, we adopted the sustained vowels /i/ in the database introduced in Sect. 4.2.2. Reliable GCI detection is critical to extracting *shimmer* (and its variants), which is a typical feature in pathological speech classification (Tsanas 2012). First, the detected GCIs are used to separate a speech into individual periods. Then the maximum amplitude in each period is gathered in a set *C* and then organized chronologically. Then *shimmer* and its variants are extracted to measure the perturbations across set *C*. The exact definitions of *shimmer* and its variants can be found in the work of Tsanas (2012). Then only *shimmer* and its variants, which are composed of 22 dimensions altogether, are adopted for classification and features uncorrelated with GCI are beyond our focus.

Table 4.4 Comparisons of GCI detection algorithms on pathological voice recognition

Method	Classification accuracy (%)	F1 measure (%)
MSM	74.08	73.58
ZFR	74.32	76.82
SEDREAMS	78.13	79.41
$GMAT_{max}$	67.74	72.17
$GMAT_{prod}$	70.62	71.27
$GMAT_{mean}$	75.08	75.82

The *shimmer* feature and its variants are highly correlated (Tsanas 2012). Hence, principal component analysis (PCA) follows the feature extraction to alleviate the correlation and to reduce the number of dimensions. The dimensions after reduction include 99.9% of the variance. Finally, the well-performing classifier Support Vector Machine (SVM) with radial basis function kernel (note that kernel functions and the corresponding parameters are tuned to obtain the best performance) is adopted for classification. Note that 60% of the samples are selected randomly for training the classifier and the remaining are for testing. The classification is repeated 100 times with randomized training and test sets and the averaged test accuracy is reported.

With different GCI detection methods, the values of *shimmer* related features and the final classification accuracies changed. Table 4.4 provides the corresponding classification accuracies when GCIs are extracted with MSM, ZFR, SEDREAMS, and MSM. Here, F1-measure (Rijsbergen 1979) is added to handle the imbalance of sample size. From this table, we find that SEDREAMS leads to the highest accuracy and F1-score. $GMAT_{prod}$ and $GMAT_{max}$ result in lower classification rates. In fact, only the maximum amplitude in each period is needed in the definition of *shimmer*. Hence, the identification rate of the GCI detection algorithm is of more importance than bias in this application. Therefore, SEDREAMS has the highest classification rate and the strength of $GMAT_{mean}$ in this practical application is witnessed.

4.5   Discussion

4.5.1   Parameter Sensitivity

There are two parameters in the GMAT algorithm, window length T_l and scale parameter M. In this section, their effects on the performance of GMAT are analyzed.

4.5.1.1   Analysis of the Scale Number M

It was stated (Khanagha et al. 2014b) that the choice of scale was crucial to the MSM method. In this experiment, the scale number ranges from 1 to 20 and four metrics

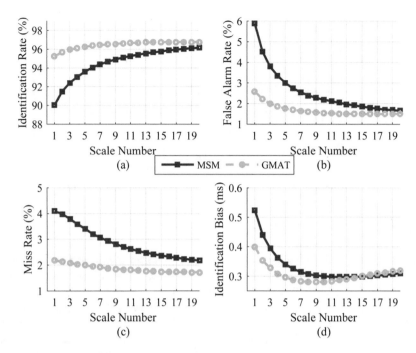

Fig. 4.10 (color online) Performance of GMAT and MSM, with the scale parameter varying from 1 to 20

are employed with IDR, MR, and FAR measuring reliability and IDB measuring accuracy. The presented result here for GMAT is averaged over the three GMAT variants. In addition, the experiments are performed on the four clean speech databases and Fig. 4.10 illustrates the comparison results.

Clearly, scale number affects the performance of GMAT and MSM. For GMAT, three reliability measurements keep almost unchanged when the scale number is over 9 and the lowest IDB is achieved with the scale number being 9. Thus, the optimal scale number for GMAT should be set to 9. In a scale-to-scale comparison, IDR of GMAT is higher than that of MSM and IDB of GMAT is lower when the scale number is less than 15. Besides, MSM is more sensitive to the scale number comparing with GMAT. In summary, GMAT is less sensitive to the choice of scale number and MSM requires a larger scale number to gain the same performance of GMAT.

4.5.1.2   Analysis of Window Length T_l

As in Eq. (4.9), window length parameter T_l is used to compute the average amplitude changes of signal $p_2(n)$. A too short window length will lead to high false alarm rate, while a too large window length may cause an increase of miss rate.

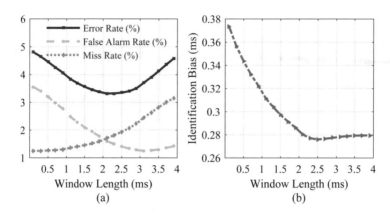

Fig. 4.11 (color online) Performance of GMAT for different window length

Therefore, the window length should be chosen appropriately to achieve the trade-off between false alarm rate and miss rate. To show the effect of window length experimentally, the applied metrics are false alarm rate (FAR), miss rate (MR), misidentification rate (it equals to FAR+MR), and the identification bias (IDB).

Figure 4.11a illustrates how misidentification rate (FAR+MR), false alarm rate (FAR), and miss rate (MR) vary with the parameter T_l. With both misidentification rate and bias taken into consideration, the window length in the proposed algorithm GMAT is set to 2.5 ms.

Based on our previous analyses, GMAT has better reliability performance than ZFR on noisy speech and it is much more accurate than ZFR on both clean and noisy speech. Even though SEDREAMS generally gives higher identification rate than GMAT on clean speech, its performance degrades greatly for noisy speech. Specially, IDR of SEDREAMS is over 10% points lower than that of GMAT in case of negative SNRs. Moreover, SEDREAMS is overwhelmingly slower than GMAT and it needs the knowledge of average pitch before detection. When it comes to the comparison between GMAT and MSM, GMAT outperforms MSM in several aspects.

- Better reliability and higher accuracy on clean speech.
- Advantageous reliability for noisy speech of 11 SNR levels (for $GMAT_{prod}$ and $GMAT_{mean}$) and nine noise types.
- Overall lower identification bias on noisy speech.
- Lower scale parameter sensitivity.
- *Lower* running time.
- Higher accuracy in pathological speech classification ($GMAT_{mean}$).

Three more issues are discussed in this section. First, we explain the reason why MSM shows better performance than GMAT, when speech is contaminated with noise type *N7* and *N11*. The second is to investigate the relation between GMAT and MSM in theory. Finally, we explain intuitively why $GMAT_{mean}$ performs better than $GMAT_{max}$ and $GMAT_{prod}$ on noisy speech.

4.5.2 GMAT and Low Frequency Noise

In Sect. 4.4, we find that GMAT based algorithms achieve better accuracy and reliability than MSM for most noise types, especially for type N2 (*destroyer engine room noise*), N6 (*high frequency radio channel noise*), and N12 (*white noise*). Nevertheless, MSM can cope with noise N7 (*military vehicle noise*) and N11 (*vehicle interior noise*) better than GMAT. In fact, noise type N7 and N11 are low frequency noises. In MSM, the scale-dependent functional is equivalent to the absolute of second derivative. Thus, slowly changing noise like N7 and N11 in noisy speech can be effectively mitigated through the derivative. For GMAT, however, the operator aTKEO is not effective for low frequency noise suppression, as analyzed below.

Let $e(n)$ denote an additive low frequency noise and $s(n)$ represent a clean speech, then the noisy speech equals to $s(n) + e(n)$. For a slowly changing noise like N7 and N11, it is reasonable to assume that $e(n-1) \approx e(n) \approx e(n+1) = \alpha$. If we denote the absolute of second derivative in MSM by an operator Γ, then $\Gamma(s(n) + e(n))$ can be approximated:

$$
\begin{aligned}
&\Gamma(s(n) + e(n)) \\
&\approx |2(s(n) + \alpha) - (s(n-1) + \alpha) - (s(n+1) + \alpha)| = \Gamma(s(n)).
\end{aligned}
\tag{4.10}
$$

Hence, low frequency noise can be dramatically reduced in MSM. In contrast, the impact of low frequency noise cannot be alleviated in GMAT since nonlinearity in the operator TKEO introduces cross-term between noise and signal. From this perspective, we interpret the comparison results for noise type N7 and N11.

4.5.3 Relation Between GMAT and MSM

The experimental results in Sect. 4.4 show that TKEO based algorithm GMAT outperforms the second derivative based method MSM. In the following, we show that the operator TKEO is linked to the local-mean-weighted second derivative. With a signal x_n, the following formulation holds:

$$
\begin{aligned}
&(x_n - (0.5x_{n-1} + 0.5x_{n+1}))(x_n + (0.5x_{n-1} + 0.5x_{n+1})) \\
&= x_n^2 - (0.5x_{n-1} + 0.5x_{n+1})^2 \\
&\leq x_n^2 - x_{n-1}x_{n+1}.
\end{aligned}
\tag{4.11}
$$

Here, $x_n - (0.5x_{n-1} + 0.5x_{n+1})$ denotes the second derivation of x_n and $x_n^2 - x_{n-1}x_{n+1}$ means the TKEO output. In addition, the term $x_n + (0.5x_{n-1} + 0.5x_{n+1})$ is the local mean. The equality in Eq. (4.11) holds if $x_{n-1} = x_{n+1}$. From this equation, operator TKEO is closely related to the local-mean-weighted second derivative.

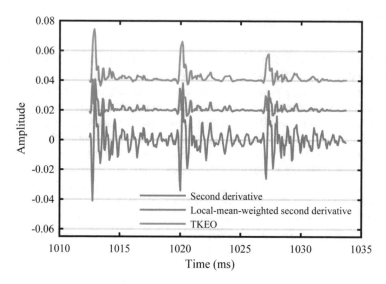

Fig. 4.12 (color online) An example showing the relation between the second derivative operator and TKEO. Note that the results of local-mean-weighted second derivative and TKEO are shifted upwards by a unit of 0.02 and 0.04 for better display

Figure 4.12 shows the result of second derivative, TKEO, and local-mean-weighted second derivative for a speech segment. For clear display, the results of local-mean-weighted second derivative and TKEO are shifted upwards by a unit of 0.02 and 0.04, respectively. Besides, GCI ground truths are added. It is observed that the second derivative result has more fluctuations in each period. The TKEO result, however, yields peaks around GCIs and tends to have low and stable amplitudes elsewhere. As in line with Eq. (4.11), the waveform of local-mean-weighted second derivative shows similarity with the TKEO result (notice that the amplitude for TKEO result is larger). Therefore, we may conclude that operator TKEO is similar to the local-mean-weighted second derivative and TKEO is more suitable for GCI detection than the second derivative due to the less fluctuating interferences. Hence, we attribute the advantages of GMAT over MSM to the effect of local-mean weighting.

4.5.4 Different Pooling Methods in GMAT

In Sect. 4.4, the performances of three GMAT based algorithms $GMAT_{max}$, $GMAT_{prod}$, and $GMAT_{mean}$ are compared. If all aspects are considered, $GMAT_{mean}$ method performs the best. While $GMAT_{prod}$ has comparable reliability and accuracy for clean and noisy speech, its running time is relatively higher. Comparing with $GMAT_{mean}$, $GMAT_{max}$ often gives lower reliability (IDR) for both clean and noisy speech. Besides, the performance of $GMAT_{max}$ is the worst among $GMAT_{max}$, $GMAT_{prod}$, and $GMAT_{mean}$ in pathological speech classification.

$GMAT_{mean}$ adopts an average pooling to fuse the results of multiscale aTKEO. Comparing with max pooling in $GMAT_{max}$ and multiscale product in $GMAT_{prod}$, average pooling is more robust to outliers and noise. Hence, $GMAT_{mean}$ will be used for our future GCI detection.

4.6 Summary

In this chapter, we present a novel GCI detection approach GMAT. In GMAT, two elements are crucial: the operator TKEO and the multiscale technique. Due to nonlinearities in speech production, the nonlinear "energy" operator TKEO is applied for GCI detection. To enhance the robustness of aTKEO indicating a GCI, three pooling techniques are used to fuse the multiscale results of aTKEO, which are max pooling, multiscale product, and mean pooling. The developed GCI detection algorithms are named as $GMAT_{max}$, $GMAT_{prod}$, and $GMAT_{mean}$, respectively. Finally, GCIs are detected using the fused results. Experiments show the advantages of GMAT: (1) lowest identification bias on clean speech; (2) highest performances for most SNR levels for noisy speech; (3) less sensitive to parameter scale number; (4) low computational cost. In addition, GMAT proves its ability in a practical application, which is pathological speech classification.

We expect that the proposed GMAT based methods, especially $GMAT_{mean}$, are helpful for GCI detection. As experiments and discussion indicate, GMAT is less competitive for speech contaminated by low frequency noise. Besides, it is interesting to investigate whether using intermediate result of GMAT can detect the voiced regions for a real speech. In the future, we may explore solutions to these issues.

References

Abu-Shikhah, N., & Deriche, M. (1999). A novel pitch estimation technique using the Teager energy function. In *International symposium on signal processing and ITS applications* (pp.135-138).

Adiga, N., & Prasanna, S. M. (2013). Significance of instants of significant excitation for source modeling. In *Proceeding of Interspeech* (pp. 1677-1681).

Adiga, N., Govind, D., & Prasanna, S. M. (2014). Significance of epoch identification accuracy for prosody modification. In *IEEE International conference on signal processing and communications* (pp.1-6).

Alku, P. (2011). Glottal inverse filtering analysis of human voice production - A review of estimation and parameterization methods of the glottal excitation and their applications. *Sadhana, 36*(5), 623-650.

Ananthapadmanabha, T., & Yegnanarayana, B. (1979). Epoch extraction from linear prediction residual for identification of closed glottis interval. *IEEE Trans. Acoust. Speech Signal Process., 27*(4), 309-319.

Bahoura, M., & Rouat, J. (2001). Wavelet speech enhancement based on the Teager Energy operator. *IEEE Signal Process. Lett., 8*(1), 10-12.

Banerjee, P. K., & Chakrabarti, N. B. (2015). Noise sensitivity of Teager-Kaiser energy operators and their ratios. In *IEEE International advances in computing, communications and informatics* (pp. 2265-2271).

Bouzid, A., & Ellouze, N. (2008). Open quotient measurements based on multiscale product of speech signal wavelet transform. *Research Lett. Signal Process.,* 1-5.

Bozkurt, B., & Dutoit, T. (2003). Mixed-phase speech modeling and formant estimation, using differential phase spectrums. In *ISCA voice quality conference* (pp. 21-24).

Brookes, M., Naylor, P. A., & Gudnason, J. (2006). A quantitative assessment of group delay methods for identifying glottal closures in voiced speech. *IEEE Trans. Audio Speech Lang. Process., 14*(2), 456-466.

Chen, S. H., Wu, H. T., Chang, Y., & Truong, T. K. (2007). Robust voice activity detection using perceptual wavelet-packet transform and Teager energy operator. *Pattern Recognit. Lett., 28* (11), 1327-1332.

Choi, J. H., & Kim, T. (2002). Neural action potential detector using multi-resolution TEO. *Electron. Lett., 38*(12), 541-543.

Choi, J. H., Jung, H. K., & Kim, T. (2006). A new action potential detector using the MTEO and its effects on spike sorting systems at low signal-to-noise ratios. *IEEE Trans. Biomed. Eng., 53*(4), 738-746.

D'Alessandro, C., & Sturmel, N. (2011). Glottal closure instant and voice source analysis using time-scale lines of maximum amplitude. *Sādhanā, 36*(5), 601-622.

Daoudi, K., & Kumar, A. J. (2015). Pitch-based speech perturbation measures using a novel GCI detection algorithm: Application to pathological voice classification. In *Proceeding of Interspeech* (pp. 3725-3728).

Drira, A., Guillon, L., & Boudraa, A. O. (2014). Image source detection for geoacoustic inversion by the Teager-Kaiser energy operator. *J. Acoust. Soc. Am., 135*(6), EL258-EL264.

Drugman, T., & Dutoit, T. (2009). Glottal closure and opening instant detection from speech signals. In *Proceeding of Interspeech* (pp. 2891-2894).

Drugman, T., Bozkurt, B., & Dutoit, T. (2011). Causal-anticausal decomposition of speech using complex cepstrum for glottal source estimation. *Speech Comm., 53*(6), 855-866.

Drugman, T., & Dutoit, T. (2011). Oscillating Statistical Moments for Speech Polarity Detection. In *Proceedings of Non-Linear Speech Processing Workshop (NOLISP11)* (pp.48–54).

Drugman, T., Thomas, M., Gudnason, J., & Naylor, P. (2012). Detection of glottal closure instants from speech signals: a quantitative review. *IEEE Trans. Audio Speech Lang. Process., 20*(3), 994-1006.

Drugman, T., Wilfart, G., & Dutoit, T. (2009). A deterministic plus stochastic model of the residual signal for improved parametric speech synthesis. In *Proceeding of Interspeech* (pp.1779-1782).

Erdamar, A., Duman, F., & Yetkin, S. (2012). A wavelet and Teager energy operator based method for automatic detection of K-Complex in sleep EEG. *Expert Syst. Appl., 39*(1), 1284-1290.

Fant, G. (1970). *Acoustic Theory of Speech Production.* Mouton, Paris.

Gaubitch, N. D., & Naylor, P. A. (2007). Spatiotemporal averaging method for enhancement of reverberant speech. In *IEEE International conference on digital signal processing* (pp. 607-610).

Guerchi, D., & Mermelstein, P. (2000). Low-rate quantization of spectral information in a 4 kb/s pitch-synchronous CELP coder. In *IEEE workshop on speech coding* (pp. 111-113).

Jabloun, F., & Cetin, A. E. (1999). The Teager energy based feature parameters for robust speech recognition in car noise. *IEEE Signal Process. Lett., 6*(10), 259-261.

Kaiser, J. F. (1990). On a simple algorithm to calculate the 'energy' of a signal. In *IEEE International conference on acoustics, speech and signal processing* (pp.381-384).

Kandali, A. B., Routray, A., & Basu, T. K. (2009). Vocal emotion recognition in five native languages of Assam using new wavelet features. *Int. J. Speech Technol., 12*(1), 1-13.

Kane, J., & Gobl, C. (2013). Evaluation of glottal closure instant detection in a range of voice qualities. *Speech Comm., 55*(2), 295-314.

Khanagha, V. (2013a). *Matlab codes for Glottal Closure Instants (GCI) detection,* Available online: http://geostat.bordeaux.inria.fr/.

Khanagha, V. (2013b). *Novel multiscale methods for nonlinear speech analysis,* Doctoral dissertation, Université Sciences et Technologies-Bordeaux I, Bordeaux.

Khanagha, V., Daoudi, K., & Yahia, H. M. (2014b). Detection of glottal closure instants based on the microcanonical multiscale formalism. *IEEE/ACM Trans. Audio Speech Lang. Process., 22* (12), 1941-1950.

Khanagha, V., Daoudi, K., Pont, O., Yahia, H., & Turiel, A. (2014a). Non-linear speech representation based on local predictability exponents. *Neurocomputing, 132*(132), 136-141.

Kominek, J., & Black, A. W. (2004). The CMU Arctic speech databases. *Proc of Isca Speech Synthesis Workshop, 99*(4), 223-224. Available online: http://festvox.org/.

Maragos, P., Kaiser, J. F., & Quatieri, T. F. (1993). Energy separation in signal modulations with application to speech analysis. *IEEE Trans. Signal Process., 41*(10), 3024-3051.

Mitra, S. K., Li, H., Lin, I. S., & Yu, T. H. (1991). A new class of nonlinear filters for image enhancement. In *IEEE International conference on acoustics, speech and signal processing* (pp. 2525-2528).

Mitra, V., Franco, H., Graciarena, M., & Mandal, A. (2012). Normalized amplitude modulation features for large vocabulary noise-robust speech recognition. In *IEEE International conference on acoustics, speech and signal processing* (pp.4117-4120).

Moulines, E., & Charpentier, F. (1990). Pitch-synchronous waveform processing techniques for text-to-speech synthesis using diphones. *Speech Comm., 9*(5–6), 453-467.

Mukhopadhyay, S., & Ray, G. C. (1998). A new interpretation of nonlinear energy operator and its efficacy in spike detection. *IEEE Trans Biomed. Eng., 45*(2), 180-187.

Murty, K. S. R., & Yegnanarayana, B. (2006). Combining evidence from residual phase and MFCC features for speaker recognition. *IEEE Signal Process. Lett., 13*(1), 52-55.

Naylor, P. A., Kounoudes, A., Gudnason, J., & Brookes, M. (2007). Estimation of glottal closure instants in voiced speech using the DYPSA algorithm. *IEEE Trans. Audio Speech Lang. Process., 15*(1), 34-43.

Nelson, R., Myers, S. M., Simonotto, J. D., Furman, M. D., Spano, M., & Norman, W. M., et al. (2006). Detection of high frequency oscillations with Teager energy in an animal model of limbic epilepsy. In *International conference of the IEEE engineering in medicine & biology society* (pp.2578-2580).

Ning, C., & Ying, H. U. (2007). Pitch detection algorithm based on Teager energy operator and spatial correlation function. In *2007 International conference on machine learning and cybernetics* (pp.2456-2460).

Pantazis, Y., Stylianou, Y., & Klabbers, E. (2005). Discontinuity detection in concatenated speech synthesis based on nonlinear speech analysis. In *Proceeding of Interspeech* (pp. 2817-2820).

Patil, H. A., & Baljekar, P. N. (2011). Novel VTEO based Mel cepstral features for classification of normal and pathological voices. In *Proceeding of Interspeech* (pp. 509-512).

Patil, H. A., & Viswanath, S. (2011). Effectiveness of Teager energy operator for epoch detection from speech signals. *Int. J. Speech Technol., 14*(4), 321-337.

Pineda-Sanchez, M., Puche-Panadero, R., Riera-Guasp, M., Perez-Cruz, J., Roger-Folch, J., & Pons-Llinares, J., et al. (2013). Application of the Teager–Kaiser energy operator to the fault diagnosis of induction motors. *IEEE Trans. Energy Conversion, 28*(4), 1036-1044.

Prathosh, A. P., Ananthapadmanabha, T. V., & Ramakrishnan, A. G. (2013). Epoch extraction based on integrated linear prediction residual using Plosion index. *IEEE Trans. Audio Speech Lang. Process., 21*(12), 2471-2480.

Rao, K. S., & Yegnanarayana, B. (2006). Prosody modification using instants of significant excitation. *IEEE Trans. Audio Speech Lang. Process.,14*(3), 972-980.

Rijsbergen, C. J. V. (1979). *Information Retrieval.* Butterworth-Heinemann.

Solnik, S., Rider, P. K., Devita, P., & Hortobagyi, T. (2010). Teager-Kaiser energy operator signal conditioning improves EMG onset detection. *Eur. J. Appl. Physiol., 110*(3), 489-498.

Rao, K. S., Prasanna, S. M., & Yegnanarayana, B. (2007). Determination of instants of significant excitation in speech using Hilbert envelope and group delay function. *IEEE Signal Process. Lett., 14*(10), 762-765.

Murty, K. S. R., & Yegnanarayana, B. (2008). Epoch extraction from speech signals. *IEEE Trans. Audio Speech Lang. Process., 16*(8), 1602-1613.

Sturmel, N., d'Alessandro, C., & Rigaud, F. (2009). Glottal closure instant detection using Lines of Maximum Amplitudes (LOMA) of the wavelet transform. In *IEEE International conference on acoustics, speech and signal processing* (pp.4517-4520).

Subasi, A., Yilmaz, A. S., & Tufan, K. (2011). Detection of generated and measured transient power quality events using Teager energy operator. *Energy Conversion & Manag., 52*(4), 1959-1967.

Teager, H. (1980). Some observations on oral air flow during phonation. *IEEE Trans. Audio Speech Lang. Process., 28*(5), 599-601.

Teager, H. M., & Teager, S. M. (1990). Evidence for nonlinear sound production mechanisms in the vocal tract. *Speech Prod. Speech Model., 55*, 241-261.

Thomas, M. R. P., Gaubitch, N. D., Gudnason, J., & Naylor, P. A. (2007). A practical multichannel dereverberation algorithm using multichannel DYPSA and spatiotemporal averaging. In *2007 IEEE workshop on applications of signal processing to audio and acoustics* (pp.50-53).

Thomas, M. R. P., Gudnason, J., & Naylor, P. A. (2009). Data-driven voice source waveform modelling. In *2014 IEEE international conference on acoustics, speech and signal processing* (pp.3965-3968).

Thomas, M. R. P., Gudnason, J., & Naylor, P. A. (2012). Estimation of glottal closing and opening instants in voiced speech using the YAGA algorithm. *IEEE Trans. Audio Speech Lang. Process., 20*(1), 82-91.

Tomar, V., & Patil, H. A. (2008). On the development of variable length Teager energy operator (VTEO). In *Proceeding of Interspeech* (pp. 1056-1059).

Tsanas, A. (2012). *Accurate telemonitoring of Parkinson's disease symptom severity using nonlinear speech signal processing and statistical machine learning.* Doctoral dissertation, Oxford University. Oxford.

Tuan, V. N., & d'Alessandro, C. (1999). Robust glottal closure detection using the wavelet transform. In *6th European conference on speech communication and technology* (pp.2805-2808).

Ulriksen, M. D., & Damkilde, L. (2016). Structural damage localization by outlier analysis of signal-processed mode shapes–Analytical and experimental validation. *Mech. Syst. Signal Process., 68*, 1-14.

Varga, A., Steeneken, H. J. M., & Jones, D. (1992). *Reports of NATO Research Study Group (RSG. 10).*

Wu, K., Zhang, D., & Lu, G. (2017). GMAT: Glottal closure instants detection based on the Multiresolution Absolute Teager–Kaiser energy operator. *Digital Signal Process., 69*, 286-299.

Yegnanarayana, B., & Murty, K. S. R. (2009). Event-based instantaneous fundamental frequency estimation from speech signals. *IEEE Trans. Audio Speech Lang. Process., 17*(4), 614-624.

Zhou, G., Hansen, J. H. L., & Kaiser, J. F. (2001). Nonlinear feature based classification of speech under stress. *IEEE Trans. Speech Audio Process., 9*(3), 201-216.

Chapter 5
Feature Learning

Abstract Detecting Parkinson's disease (PD) based on voice analysis is meaningful due to the non-invasion and convenience. Traditional features adopted for PD detection are often hand-crafted, in which special expertise is needed. In this chapter, we propose to employ a feature learning technique to learn features automatically, where special expertise is unnecessary. First, calculate the first derivative of Mel-spectrogram with respect to time for preprocessed audio signals. Then, we use spherical K-means to train two dictionaries using samples of PD patients and healthy controls, respectively. Third, frames in an audio signal are encoded with the two dictionaries, followed by a pooling method to summarize over frames. In comparison with hand-crafted features, experiments show that the proposed method reaches higher performance in terms of four metrics. Additionally, issues like clustering number in spherical K-means and pooling method are discussed. Finally, by analyzing the similarities between the hand-crafted and learned features, some knowledge is obtained, which can guide future learning and design of features in PD detection.

Keywords Feature learning · Mel-spectrogram · Parkinson's disease · Spherical K-means

5.1 Introduction

Parkinson's disease (PD) is a slowly progressive disorder of the central nervous system. In 2016, there were about 6.06 million people worldwide affected with PD (Vos et al. 2017) and PD is the second most common neurodegenerative disorder after Alzheimer's disease. PD impairs patients' motor and cognitive functions, and even leads to death. It was reported that 211.3 thousands of people died of PD in 2016 (Mohsen et al. 2017). Up until now, there is no cure for PD, although some treatments can help to alleviate symptoms and slow down progression (Connolly and Lang 2014). Therefore, it is significant to explore the early diagnosis of PD to improve the life quality of PD patients and prolong their lives (Pereira et al. 2016).

© Springer Nature Singapore Pte Ltd. 2020
D. Zhang, K. Wu, *Pathological Voice Analysis*,
https://doi.org/10.1007/978-981-32-9196-6_5

PD patients is characterized by tremor, rigidity, slowness of movement, and gait disturbances (Sveinbjornsdottir 2016). Besides, non-motor symptoms also occur, such as sleep disorders, depression, and anxiety. Particularly, vocal impairment is present in a majority of patients with PD (PWP) (Ho et al. 1998; Chen et al. 2016), and it may be one of the earliest symptoms to diagnose PD (Harel et al. 2004; Duffy 2013). Once affected with PD, all dimensions of the speech production may be affected, such as articulation, phonation, prosody, and speech fluency (Darley et al. 1969). Common vocal symptoms include harshness, breathiness, reduced voice intensity, monopitch, disturbed speech rate, and palilalia (Brabenec et al. 2017; Little et al. 2009).

Detecting PD by acoustical analysis is user-friendly since voice recording is non-invasive and convenient. In this chapter, features used for acoustical analysis based PD detection are discussed and the organization is as follows: Section 5.2 introduces the related works on hand-crafted features and feature learning for PD detection. Section 5.3 presents details of our proposed feature learning method, followed by experimental results and discussions in Sect. 5.4. In Sect. 5.5, we summarize the chapter and present the future work.

5.2   Related Works

In PD detection, both running speech and sustained vowels have been used to assess the vocal impairment for PWP. For running speech, subjects are required to speak a pre-devised sentence containing representative linguistic units (Orozco-Arroyave et al. 2016). In terms of sustained vowels, subjects will pronounce a standard vowel of normal pitch and sustain it as long as possible (Tsanas et al. 2014; Tsanas et al. 2010). In comparison, running speech can be used to assess three dimensions of vocal impairment: phonation, articulation, and prosody, whereas vowels are mainly limited to evaluating the phonation aspect (Orozco-Arroyave et al. 2016). However, phonation and articulation in running speech are coupled together with confounding effects, making it complex to analyze. Besides, evidence showed that analyzing vowels were sufficient for PD detection (Tsanas et al. 2014; Tsanas et al. 2010). Hence, we choose to utilize sustained vowels for PD detection in this chapter.

There have been varieties of acoustical features for PD detection. In the first category, the features developed are to quantify the extent of periodicity based on the observation that vocal folds vibration in pathological voice is more likely to deviate from periodicity or is even completely aperiodic (Titze and Martin 1998). Jitter (fundamental frequency perturbation) and shimmer (amplitude perturbation over periods) are the two most representative features in this group (Tsanas 2012a). Note that there is no unique mathematical definition of jitter and shimmer, and one can find the most widely used variants in Tsanas (2012a). GQ (glottal quotient) (Tsanas 2012a) describes the deviation of time duration when the glottis is open (closed) in each glottis cycle. In Little et al. (2007), a novel measure RPDE (recurrence period density entropy) was proposed by modeling the vocal production as a nonlinear dynamical system and this measure is based on a generalization of periodicity, namely recurrence (Kantz and Schreiber 2004) which was defined as the amount of time before a segment of speech is within a constant from another segment of speech forward in time. Due to the increased uncertainty in the period of the speech signal, pathological voice typically causes an increase in RPDE. PPE (pitch period entropy) characterizes the pitch stability using a logarithmic scale, and it was demonstrated to be robust to many confounding effects (Little et al. 2009). The second group of features assesses the noise extent in voice, which is often caused by incomplete glottal closure and shown with symptoms like breathiness and harshness. HNR (harmonics-to-noise ratio) and NHR (noise-to-harmonics ratio) are classic features in this category and their variants can be found in Ferrer et al. (2006). DFA (detrended fluctuation analysis) (Little et al. 2007) is devised based on the nonlinear dynamic theory to quantify the extent of turbulent noise in the vocal tract. Glottal-to-noise excitation (GNE), vocal fold excitation ratio (VFER), and empirical mode decomposition excitation ratio (EMD-ER) are also measures to quantify the increased acoustic noise (Tsanas 2012a). In the third class, features devised for speech and speaker recognition are included. For instance, it was evidenced that MFCC (Mel-frequency cepstral coefficients), together with its first and second derivatives in time (over successive frames), were effective to detect PD (Naranjo et al. 2016; Vasquez-Correa et al. 2015; Mekyska et al. 2016; Bocklet et al. 2011) and predict PD severity (Tsanas 2012a). The discrimination power of LPC (linear prediction coefficients) and LPCC (linear prediction cepstral coefficients) for PD detection was analyzed (Mekyska et al. 2016; Orozco-Arroyave et al. 2013). A study in Mekyska et al. (2016) even indicated that features such as LPC, LPCC, and MFCC outperformed conventional ones for PD detection despite their low clinical interpretability. More widely used features can be found in Mekyska et al. (2015). Several publicly available tools are developed to calculate these features: PRAAT (Boersma and Weenink 2009) and MDVP (Multi-Dimensional Voice Program) (Elemetrics 2012) provide calculation of several classical features; VOICEBOX (Brookes 2012) consists of routines for LPC, LPCC, and MFCC; Voice Analysis Toolbox (Tsanas 2012b) presents MATLAB source code for plenty of features, such as GQ, HNR, NHR, variants of jitter and shimmer, and RPDE. In Tsanas (2012a), 318-dimension hand-crafted features were extracted for the purpose of discriminating healthy controls from people with Parkinson's disease. In addition, feature selection was adopted to analyze the discriminative power of each feature and the experimental results indicated that MFCC (and its derivatives), HNR, VFER, Shimmer, and GNE were some of the effective features for PD detection. For more comparison among features, one may find the details in Tsanas (2012a) and Tsanas et al. (2014).

It is worthwhile to note that most existing features for PD detection are hand-crafted. Recently, studies especially in the field of computer vision (Krizhevsky et al. 2012; Guo et al. 2016) have witnessed the success of feature learning over manually designed features in terms of classification accuracy. In audio classification tasks, such as speech recognition (Siniscalchi et al. 2013), music information retrieval (Dieleman and Schrauwen 2013; Hamel et al. 2011; Vaizman et al. 2014), environmental sound classification (Salamon and Bello 2015a, b), and speech emotion recognition (Huang et al. 2015), feature learning technique has also shown its capacity. Comparing with traditional feature extraction, feature learning is advantageous in two aspects. First, feature learning is performed for each task so that the learned features are task-specific. Since designing feature is expensive due to the requirement of expertise, it is common that one type of hand-crafted feature is used for multiple tasks. Evidently, sharing the same feature for different tasks is not optimally effective. Second, learned feature is likely to be robust to irrelevant factors. It was argued in Salamon and Bello (2015b) that learned feature is more robust to speaker variation in the task of speech emotion recognition. While it is known that tuning parameters in feature learning with deep layers can be challenging, there have been researches showing that simple feature learning approach with few parameters can also be impressively competitive, sometimes even better than methods based on deep layers (Coates et al. 2011). As an example, spherical K-means with a single parameter was proved to be a simple but powerful approach to learn feature (Dieleman and Schrauwen 2013; Salamon and Bello 2015a, b; Coates et al. 2011). Hence, we are motivated to investigate feature learning technique for PD detection so that features with high discrimination power and robustness to factors like speaker variation can be obtained.

Unlike previous works that extract hand-crafted features, we propose to use the feature learning technique to provide features for PD detection in this chapter. Two dictionaries are learned by using spherical K-means clustering on the derivative of Mel-spectrogram (across successive frames) for PD and HC (healthy control) group, respectively. Followed by encoding and pooling, the learned features for a given voice sample can be calculated. Based on the experimental results, useful knowledge is acquired to guide feature devising and learning for PD detection in the future.

5.3   Proposed Feature Learning Method

The pipeline for our proposed method is shown in Fig. 5.1 and each included step is explained in detail below. The abbreviations in Fig. 5.1 are also expanded in the following.

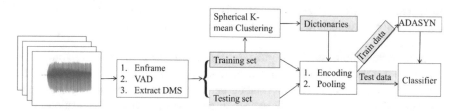

Fig. 5.1 (color online) System pipeline (blocks filled with gray color represent data and unfilled ones mean operation steps)

5.3.1   *Preprocessing*

Given a voice sample, it is first split into overlapping frames due to the property of short-time stationarity. Here, the window type used is Hamming and the frame length and inter-frame time increment are set as 50 ms and 25 ms, respectively. Then VAD (voice activity detection) is implemented to remove the unvoiced portion by the detector proposed in Martin (2001). The segmented voiced part is passed to the following steps.

5.3.2   *Mel-Spectrogram*

As demonstrated (Naranjo et al. 2016; Vasquez-Correa et al. 2015; Mekyska et al. 2016; Bocklet et al. 2011; Tsanas 2012a), MFCCs play an important role in PD detection. It is reasonable to assume that Mel-spectrogram is suitable to represent a voice signal for feature learning. For each segmented frame, its Mel-spectrogram is computed by mapping the spectral magnitudes of short-time Fourier transform onto the perceptually motivated Mel-scale using the filter bank technique (O'shaughnessy 1987). In this chapter, the number of filters in filter bank is set as 64 with the implementation in VOICEBOX. The mapping from frequency (denoted as f) to Mel-frequency (denoted as $\text{Mel}(f)$) can be expressed as below.

$$\text{Mel}(f) = 2595 \log_{10}\left(1 + \frac{f}{700}\right). \tag{5.1}$$

As implied in the physical definition of features jitter and shimmer, perturbation across time is meaningful when it comes to disorder assessment. Inspired by this observation, we then compute the first derivative of Mel-spectrogram across successive frames after obtaining the Mel-spectrograms for all frames. While Mel-spectrograms contain quantities of biometric information (as evidenced in the importance of MFCCs to speaker recognition), we argue that taking the derivative of Mel-spectrogram with respect to time alleviates the influence of speaker variation on PD detection and highlights the biomedical attributes of the given voice sample. Hereafter, the first derivative of Mel-spectrogram is abbreviated as DMS. Finally, all DMSs are stacked together as a matrix A of size $64 \times m$ to form a representation for a given voice signal, where $m + 1$ is the number of frames in this voiced segment. Note that m may vary with different voice samples.

5.3.3   *Dictionary Learning Based on Spherical K-Means*

Spherical K-means is a modified version of the traditional clustering method K-means. The main difference is that centroids in spherical K-means are required to have a unit l_2-norm (in other words, they lie on a unit sphere). Experimental evidence in Coates and Ng (2012) showed that the centroids of spherical K-means were relatively sparse projections of the data for clustering. Besides, feature learning based on spherical K-means has advantages of speed and scalability, with successful examples in the field of image recognition (O'shaughnessy 1987) and audio classification (Dieleman and Schrauwen 2013; Hamel et al. 2011; Vaizman et al. 2014; Salamon and Bello 2015a, b; Huang et al. 2015). Therefore, spherical K-means is utilized for dictionary learning. Suppose a data matrix is represented by $V \in R^{l \times n}$, then the routines for spherical K-means can be implemented by iterating the followings until convergence:

$$s_j^{(i)} := \begin{cases} D^{(j)\mathrm{T}}v^{(i)}, \text{if } j == \arg\max_w \mid D^{(w)\mathrm{T}}v^{(i)} \mid, \forall i,j. \\ 0, \hspace{4.5cm} \text{otherwise} \end{cases} \tag{5.2}$$

$$D := VS^\mathrm{T} + D. \tag{5.3}$$

$$D^{(j)} := D^{(j)} / \left\| D^{(j)} \right\|_2, \forall j. \tag{5.4}$$

where D is the learned codebook of k atoms and T indicates matrix transposition. $s^{(i)}$ denotes the code vector associated with sample $v^{(i)}$ and it is the ith column in matrix S. For more detailed information on spherical K-means, one may refer to the work (Coates and Ng 2012).

Following the pipeline in Fig. 5.1, we use spherical K-means to learn two dictionaries for PD and HC classes separately. First, the DMS matrices obtained in Sect. 5.3.2 for all PD (HC) samples in the training set are stacked together for normalization and ZCA (zero component analysis) whitening to remove the correlations between different bands. Then spherical K-means is applied for clustering and the obtained centroids are regarded as atoms in the learned dictionary D_p (D_h). Let us denote the clustering number in spherical K-means as k, the learned codebook D_p (D_h) for PD (HC) group will have the size of $64 \times k$. The effect of parameter k will be optimized and discussed in Sect. 5.4.

5.3.4   *Encoding and Pooling*

In Sect. 5.3.2, a voice sample (no matter it is in the training or testing set) is represented by a matrix A consisting of stacked DMSs. In this section, the matrix is encoded with the learned dictionaries D_p and D_h to obtain the learned features.

The simple yet effective linear coding scheme (Dieleman and Schrauwen 2013; Salamon and Bello 2015b) is applied. In detail, we first multiply the matrix A by the learned dictionaries $D_p{}^T$ and $D_h{}^T$, respectively. Then the resulting two products are concatenated vertically into a matrix E, as expressed in Eq. (5.5).

$$E = \left[D_p{}^T \times A; D_h{}^T \times A \right]. \tag{5.5}$$

Next, pooling technique is used to summarize columns in E into a column vector x, where x is regarded as the learned feature with the dimension of $2k$. Some possible pooling operations include mean, standard deviation, maximum, and minimum (Hamel et al. 2011). In Sect. 5.4.3, these four pooling methods are compared in terms of performance in PD detection. With all steps together, the proposed method represents a given sample with the learned feature: a $2k$-dimensional vector.

5.4 Experimental Results

5.4.1 Dataset and Experimental Setup

Using the same voice acquisition system introduced in Sect. 2.2, the sample size of patients with PD and healthy subjects is increased to 139 and 446, respectively, when this work began. To verify the effectiveness of the proposed feature learning algorithm, the sustained vowels /i:/ with a normal pitch are used. For detailed information about experimental setting and results in this part, one can refer to the literature (Wu et al. 2018).

Clearly, the task of PD detection here is characterized by class imbalance since the number of PD is far less than that of healthy subjects. Re-sampling is one of the most widely used methods (Cateni et al. 2014) to deal with class imbalance. For instance, experimental results in Lopez et al. (2013) proved the good performances of ADASYN (adaptive synthetic sampling). It uses a weighted distribution of minority samples (PD) to decide the number of synthetic samples that are to be generated for each minority sample. In this way, lots of synthetic samples are generated near the minority side of the classification decision boundary. Adding the synthetic samples generated by ADASYN to the minority class compensates for the skewed distributions and the distribution of the resulting dataset will be more balanced. Note that the synthetic samples are used for training only. For more detailed descriptions of the ADASYN algorithm, readers may refer to He et al. (2008).

Accuracy rate (*Acc*) is not enough in the occasion of class imbalanced dataset since it cannot distinguish between the numbers of correctly classified examples of different classes. Therefore, three other metrics aside from accuracy rate are used, which are sensitivity (*Sen*), specificity (*Spe*), and the geometric mean (*Gmean*) of *Sen* and *Spe*. The metric *Gmean* is added due to class imbalance. More discussions

Table 5.1 Confusion matrix
for a two-class problem

	PD prediction	HC prediction
PD class	True positive (TP)	False negative (FN)
HC class	False positive (FP)	True negative (TN)

on the metrics for imbalanced data can be found in Lopez et al. (2013). Table 5.1 shows the confusion matrix recording the results of correctly and incorrectly recognized instances of each class, where positive and negative classes refer to PD and HC classes, respectively. The four employed metrics are defined by Eqs. (5.6)–(5.9).

$$\text{Acc} = \frac{TP + TN}{TP + FN + FP + TN}. \tag{5.6}$$

$$\text{Sen} = \frac{TP}{TP + FN} \tag{5.7}$$

$$\text{Spe} = \frac{TN}{FP + TN}. \tag{5.8}$$

$$\text{Gmean} = \sqrt{\frac{TP}{TP + FN} \times \frac{TN}{FP + TN}}. \tag{5.9}$$

In the proposed feature learning algorithm, the clustering number of spherical K-means is set to 16. The operation used for pooling is maximum. At the beginning of dictionary training, samples in the dataset are split into training and testing samples with a threefold cross-validation. Specially, we point out that (1) the splitting is performed for two classes separately; (2) the training indices of each class for dictionary training are the same for training classifiers. The process after extracting DMS is repeated 5 times and the averaged performance is reported. The performance of typical hand-crafted features is presented as a baseline to compare with our learned features. The 138-dimensional engineered features include (number in brackets stands for the dimensionality): variants of jitter (22), variants of shimmer (22), statistics of HNR (2) and NHR (2), GQ related (3), MFCC related (84), DFA (1), RPDE (1), and PPE (1). All these features are defined in Tsanas (2012a) and can be computed using Matlab routines in the Voice Analysis Toolbox with parameters set as default (Tsanas 2012b). Similarly, threefold cross-validation in the classification stage is employed and repeated 5 times, within which synthetic samples are generated by ADASYN for each training set separately.

5.4.2   PD Detection with Learned and Hand-Crafted Features

In comparison, feature selection is added so that optimal performance can be obtained for both types of features. Even though feature selection methods are broadly categorized into three groups (Chandrashekar and Sahin 2014): the filter, wrapper, and embedded methods, we adopt one of the simplest filter methods, which is correlation criteria, to select features. The optimal number of selected features is determined when the average *Gmean* reaches its maximum. Random forest (RF) and linear SVM are adopted for classification because of their good performances in plentiful of comparisons (Fernandez-Delgado et al. 2014).

The performances of learned and hand-crafted features are shown in Table 5.2. First, it turns out that SVM works better for hand-crafted features, whereas learned features have better performance with RF classifier. Second, comparing with hand-crafted features, learned features achieve higher *Acc*, *Gmean*, *Sen*, and *Spe*. Third, detecting PD with learned features is more stable since the standard derivation with four metrics is all lower. Therefore, we may conclude that the proposed feature learning algorithm for PD detection outperforms the traditional hand-crafted features. The reasons behind may be highly related with the property of task-specific feature learning, which can learn the real acoustic differences between PD and HC group. Besides, the encoded features with the union of two dictionaries learnt separately can be more predictive.

When using learned features to detect PD, we notice that the highest sensitivity is around 82%, while the highest specificity is nearly 93%. Class imbalance is likely to be responsible for the rate difference, even though ADASYN strategy is used. In addition, there is an interesting finding that nine of the top ten features in the ranked hand-crafted feature set to come from the MFCC related features, which further validates the rationality to choose Mel-spectrum for the proposed feature learning to discriminate PD patients and HC.

5.4.3 Ablation Study

5.4.3.1 Clustering Number in Spherical K-Means

Clustering number is a key parameter in spherical K-means. If the clustering number is too small, the learned dictionaries cannot fully characterize the acoustic difference between PD and HC. On the other hand, if the number of clusters is too large, training dictionaries will be more time-consuming and the atoms in dictionaries are highly correlated with each other, which brings litter improvement and sometimes even hinders PD detection.

In this section, we design an experiment to gain insights into its effect on the performance of PD detection by setting clustering number k as $\{4; 8; 16; 32; 64\}$. Maximum pooling is adopted and feature selection is no longer implemented. Two metrics are adopted for evaluations here: *Acc* and *Gmean*, which is a metric balancing *Sen* and *Spe*. The classifier used is RF since it is indicated in the above experiment that RF works better for the proposed features than SVM.

Figure 5.2 illustrates the results of comparison. With both performance and running time into considerations, the clustering number in our proposed algorithm is set to 32.

Table 5.2 Performance of hand-crafted and learned features in PD detection

Feature	Clf	Acc (%)	Gmean (%)	Sen (%)	Spe (%)
Crafted	SVM	**79.44 ± 3.25**	**73.56 ± 3.92**	64.69 ± 6.89	**84.00 ± 4.31**
	RF	77.89 ± 3.59	72.81 ± 4.37	**65.31 ± 8.63**	81.78 ± 5.29
Learned	SVM	78.61 ± 3.11	78.60 ± 3.13	**82.09 ± 2.76**	75.38 ± 5.69
	RF	**86.17 ± 1.59**	**85.48 ± 1.68**	78.33 ± 4.19	**93.45 ± 3.69**

Bold values indicate better results

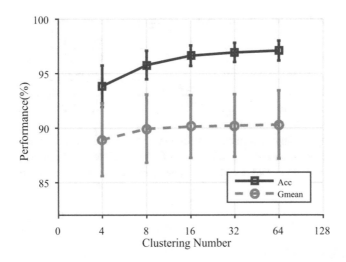

Fig. 5.2 (color online) The effect of clustering number on PD detection

Table 5.3 Performance of PD detection by different pooling methods

	Mean	Std	Maximum	Minimum
Acc	85.74 ± 1.47	84.50 ± 1.61	83.86 ± 2.10	**86.01 ± 1.58**
Gmean	85.31 ± 1.47	84.37 ± 1.56	83.07 ± 2.30	**85.33 ± 1.66**

Bold values indicate better results

Table 5.4 Shaffer test for the pooling techniques using the *Acc* metric

	Mean	Std	Maximum	Minimum
Mean	x	+(2.97e−3)	+(1.04e−6)	=(0.885)
Std	−(2.97e−3)	x	=(0.293)	−(1.59e−4)
Maximum	−(1.04e−6)	=(0.293)	x	−(1.9e−8)
Minimum	=(0.885)	+(1.59e−4)	+(1.9e−8)	x

5.4.3.2 Pooling Methods

Mean, standard deviation, maximum, and minimum are four pooling methods. Here we compare their performances in our proposed method. In the experiment, the clustering number is set to 32 and two metrics *Acc* and *Gmean* are used. As in Sect. 5.4.2, the classifier used is RF.

In Table 5.3, it is clear that minimum pooling is only advantageous over mean pooling by a narrow margin, and the maximum pooling method performs the worst since it not only has the lowest *Acc* and *Gmean*, and but also has highest deviations.

In addition, we carry out a Shaffer post-hoc test (Shaffer 1986) with the significance level set to 0.05. Consistent with the observations from Table 5.3, we find that mean and minimum pooling obtain better performances than the other two pooling methods (Table 5.4). Additionally there is no significant difference between mean

Table 5.5 Shaffer test for the pooling techniques using the *Gmean* metric

	Mean	Std	Maximum	Minimum
Mean	x	=(0.0582)	+(1.7e−8)	=(1.0)
Std	=(0.0582)	x	+(2.94e−3)	−(0.0492)
Maximum	−(1.7e−8)	−(2.94e−3)	x	−(1.27e−8)
Minimum	=(1.0)	+(0.0492)	+(1.27e−8)	x

and minimum pooling as well as between maximum and standard deviation pooling. When the metric *Gmean* is applied, the Shaffer test is shown in Table 5.5, with which the same conclusions can be drawn. Hence, either mean or minimum should be applied.

5.5   Summary

In this chapter, we propose a feature learning algorithm to learn features for PD detection automatically. To begin with, the first derivatives of Mel-spectrum were extracted and then used to train two dictionaries by spherical K-means for PD and HC groups, respectively. Finally, linear encoding together with pooling follows to obtain the learned features. In comparison with typical hand-crafted features, experiments show that the learned features got from the proposed algorithm achieve higher *Acc*, *Gmean*, *Sen*, *Spe* and lower standard derivations for the four metrics. Besides, discussion on clustering number optimization and comparisons of four different pooling method are presented.

Three representative observations drawn from this chapter are:

1. Comparing with hand-crafted features, the proposed learned features can reach higher accuracy and robustness in PD detection.
2. Mean and minimum pooling outperform maximum and standard derivation pooling.
3. Features measuring perturbation on Mel-spectrum are often useful for PD detection.

These observations will be helpful when learning and devising new features for PD detection. Besides, our algorithm provides motivation to explore feature learning technique for detecting pathological voice of other diseases. In the future, we may study the Mel-spectrum further so that the frequency bands useful for PD detection can be identified. Other future works include investigation of more effective coding scheme and fusion of pooling strategies.

References

Bocklet, T., Noth, E., Stemmer, G., Ruzickova, H., & Rusz, J. (2011). Detection of persons with Parkinson's disease by acoustic, vocal, and prosodic analysis. In *Automatic Speech Recognition and Understanding (ASRU), 2011 IEEE Workshop on* (pp. 478–483). IEEE.

Boersma, P., & Weenink, D. (2009). Praat: doing phonetics by computer (version 5.1. 12) [computer program].

Brabenec, L., Mekyska, J., Galaz, Z., & Rektorova, I. (2017). Speech disorders in Parkinson's disease: early diagnostics and effects of medication and brain stimulation. *J. Neural Transm.*, *124*, 303–334.

Brookes, M. (2012). VOICEBOX: Speech processing toolbox for MATLAB. http://www.ee.ic.ac.uk/hp/staff/dmb/voicebox/voicebox.html.

Cateni, S., Colla, V., & Vannucci, M. (2014). A method for resampling imbalanced datasets in binary classification tasks for real-world problems. *Neurocomputing*, *135*, 32–41.

Chandrashekar, G., & Sahin, F. (2014). A survey on feature selection methods. *Comput. Electr. Eng.*, *40*, 16–28.

Chen, H. L., Wang, G., Ma, C., Cai, Z. N., Liu, W. B., & Wang, S. J. (2016). An efficient hybrid kernel extreme learning machine approach for early diagnosis of Parkinson's disease. *Neurocomputing*, *184*, 131 – 144.

Coates, A., Ng, A., & Lee, H. (2011). An analysis of single-layer networks in unsupervised feature learning. In *Proceedings of the fourteenth international conference on artificial intelligence and statistics* (pp. 215–223).

Coates, A., & Ng, A. Y. (2012). Learning feature representations with k-means. In *Neural networks: Tricks of the trade* (pp. 561–580). Springer.

Connolly, B. S., & Lang, A. E. (2014). Pharmacological treatment of Parkinson disease: a review. *Jama*, *311*, 1670–1683.

Darley, F. L., Aronson, A. E., & Brown, J. R. (1969). Clusters of deviant speech dimensions in the dysarthrias. *J. Speech Hear. Res.*, *12*, 462.

Dieleman, S., & Schrauwen, B. (2013). Multiscale approaches to music audio feature learning. In *14th International Society for Music Information Retrieval Conference (ISMIR-2013)* (pp. 116–121). Pontificia Universidade Catolica do Parana.

Duffy, J. R. (2013). *Motor Speech Disorders-E-Book: Substrates, Differential Diagnosis, and Management*. Elsevier Health Sciences.

Elemetrics, K. (2012). Multi-dimensional voice program (MDVP) [computer program].

Fernandez-Delgado, M., Cernadas, E., Barro, S., & Amorim, D. (2014). Do we need hundreds of classifiers to solve real world classification problems. *J. Mach. Learn. Res.*, *15*, 3133–3181.

Ferrer, C. A., Eduardo, G., & María, E. (2006). Evaluation of time and frequency domain-based methods for the estimation of harmonics-to-noise-ratios in voice signals. *Lecture Notes in Computer Science*, *4225*, 406-415.

Guo, Y., Oerlemans, A., Oerlemans, A., Lao, S., Wu, S., & Lew, M. S. (2016). Deep learning for visual understanding. *Neurocomputing*, *187*, 27–48.

Hamel, P., Lemieux, S., Bengio, Y., & Eck, D. (2011). Temporal pooling and multiscale learning for automatic annotation and ranking of music audio. In *ISMIR* (pp. 729–734).

Harel, B., Cannizzaro, M., & Snyder, P. J. (2004). Variability in fundamental frequency during speech in prodromal and incipient Parkinson's disease: A longitudinal case study. *Brain. Cogn.*, *56*, 24 – 29.

He, H., Bai, Y., Garcia, E. A., & Li, S. (2008). ADASYN: Adaptive synthetic sampling approach for imbalanced learning. In *Neural Networks, 2008. IJCNN 2008. (IEEE World Congress on Computational Intelligence). IEEE International Joint Conference on* (pp. 1322–1328). IEEE.

Ho, A. K., Iansek, R., Marigliani, C., Bradshaw, J. L., & Gates, S. (1998). Speech impairment in a large sample of patients with Parkinson's disease. *Behav. Neurol.*, *11*, 131–137.

Huang, Z., Xue, W., & Mao, Q. (2015). Speech emotion recognition with unsupervised feature learning. *Front. Inform. Technol. Elect. Eng.*, *16*, 358–366.

Kantz, H., & Schreiber T. (2004). Nonlinear time series analysis, Cambridge University Press, 2nd edition.

Krizhevsky, A., Sutskever, I., & Hinton, G. E. (2012). ImageNet classification with deep convolutional neural networks. In *Advances in neural information processing systems* (pp. 1097–1105).

Little, M. A., Mcsharry, P. E., Hunter, E. J., Spielman, J. L., & Ramig, L. O. (2009). Suitability of dysphonia measurements for telemonitoring of Parkinson's disease. *IEEE Trans. Biomed. Eng.*, *56*, 1015–1022.

Little, M. A., McSharry, P. E., Roberts, S. J., Costello, D. A., & Moroz, I. M. (2007). Exploiting nonlinear recurrence and fractal scaling properties for voice disorder detection. *Biomed. Eng. Online*, *6*, 23.

Lopez, V., Fernandez, A., Garcia, S., Palade, V., & Herrera, F. (2013). An insight into classification with imbalanced data: Empirical results and current trends on using data intrinsic characteristics. *Inf. Sci.*, *250*, 113 – 141.

Martin, R. (2001). Noise power spectral density estimation based on optimal smoothing and minimum statistics. *IEEE Trans. Speech Audio Process.*, *9*, 504–512.

Mekyska, J., Janousova, E., Gomez-Vilda, P., Smekal, Z., Rektorova, I., Eliasova, I., Kostalova, M., Mrackova, M., Alonso-Hernandez, J. B., Faundez-Zanuy, M. et al. (2015). Robust and complex approach of pathological speech signal analysis. *Neurocomputing*, *167*, 94–111.

Mekyska, J., Smekal, Z., Galaz, Z., Mzourek, Z., Rektorova, I., FaundezZanuy, M., & Lopez-de Ipina, K. (2016). Perceptual features as markers of Parkinson's disease: the issue of clinical interpretability. In *Recent Advances in Nonlinear Speech Processing* (pp. 83–91). Springer.

Mohsen, N., Alemu, A. A., Cristiana, A., M, A. K., Foad, A.-A., & *et al.* (2017). Global, regional, and national age-sex specific mortality for 264 causes of death, 1980–2016: a systematic analysis for the global burden of disease study 2016. *Lancet*, *390*, 1151–1210.

Naranjo, L., Perez, C. J., Campos-Roca, Y., & Martin, J. (2016). Addressing voice recording replications for Parkinson's disease detection. *Expert Syst. Appl.*, *46*, 286–292.

Orozco-Arroyave, J., Honig, F., Arias-Londono, J., Vargas-Bonilla, J., Daqrouq, K., Skodda, S., Rusz, J., & Noth, E. (2016). Automatic detection of Parkinson's disease in running speech spoken in three different languages. *J. Acoust. Soc. Am.*, *139*, 481–500.

Orozco-Arroyave, J. R., Arias-Londoo, J. D., Vargas-Bonilla, J. F., & Nth, E. (2013). *Perceptual Analysis of Speech Signals from People with Parkinson's Disease*. Springer Berlin Heidelberg.

O'shaughnessy, D. (1987). *Speech communication: human and machine*. Universities press.

Pereira, C. R., Weber, S. A., Hook, C., Rosa, G. H., & Papa, J. P. (2016). Deep learning-aided Parkinson's disease diagnosis from handwritten dynamics. In *Graphics, Patterns and Images (SIBGRAPI), 2016 29th SIBGRAPI Conference on* (pp. 340–346). IEEE.

Salamon, J., & Bello, J. P. (2015a). Feature learning with deep scattering for urban sound analysis. In *Signal Processing Conference (EUSIPCO), 2015 23rd European* (pp. 724–728). IEEE.

Salamon, J., & Bello, J. P. (2015b). Unsupervised feature learning for urban sound classification. In *Acoustics, Speech and Signal Processing (ICASSP), 2015 IEEE International Conference on* (pp. 171–175). IEEE.

Shaffer, J. P. (1986). Modified sequentially rejective multiple test procedures. *J. Am. Stat. Assoc.*, *81*, 826–831.

Siniscalchi, S. M., Yu, D., Deng, L., & Lee, C. H. (2013). Exploiting deep neural networks for detection-based speech recognition. *Neurocomputing*, *106*, 148–157.

Sveinbjornsdottir, S. (2016). The clinical symptoms of Parkinson's disease. *J. Neurochem.*, *139*, 318–324.

Titze, I. R., & Martin, D. W. (1998). Principles of voice production. *J. Acoust. Soc. Am.*, *104*, 1148–1148.

Tsanas, A. (2012a). *Accurate telemonitoring of Parkinson's disease symptom severity using nonlinear speech signal processing and statistical machine learning*. Ph.D. thesis University of Oxford.

Tsanas, A. (2012b). Voice analysis toolbox (version 1.0). http://people.maths.ox.ac.uk/tsanas/ software.html.

Tsanas, A., Little, M. A., Fox, C., & Ramig, L. O. (2014). Objective automatic assessment of rehabilitative speech treatment in Parkinson's disease. *IEEE Trans. Neural Syst. Rehabil. Eng.*, *22*, 181–190.

Tsanas, A., Little, M. A., McSharry, P. E., & Ramig, L. O. (2010). Accurate telemonitoring of Parkinson's disease progression by noninvasive speech tests. *IEEE Trans. Biomed. Eng.*, *57*, 884–893.

Vaizman, Y., McFee, B., & Lanckriet, G. (2014). Codebook-based audio feature representation for music information retrieval. *IEEE/ACM Trans. Audio Speech Lang. Process.*, *22*, 1483–1493.

Vasquez-Correa, J. C., Arias-Vergara, T., Orozco-Arroyave, J. R., VargasBonilla, J., Arias-Londono, J. D., & Noth, E. (2015). Automatic detection of Parkinson's disease from continuous speech recorded in non-controlled noise conditions. In *Sixteenth Annual Conference of the International Speech Communication Association*.

Wu, K., Zhang, D., Lu, G., & Guo, Z. (2018). Learning acoustic features to detect Parkinson's disease. *Neurocomputing.*, *318(87)*, 102–108.

Vos, T., Abajobir, A. A., Abbafati, C., Abbas, K. M., Abate, K. H., & *et al.* (2017). Global, regional, and national incidence, prevalence, and years lived with disability for 328 diseases and injuries for 195 countries, 1990–2016: a systematic analysis for the global burden of disease study 2016. *Lancet, 390*, 1211–1259.

Chapter 6
Joint Learning for Voice Based Disease Detection

Abstract Voice analysis provides a non-invasive way for disease detection, in which most methods only consider a single audio, although different audios contain complementary information and a fusion of them is beneficial. In this chapter, a novel model JOLL4R (JOint Learning based on Label Relaxed low-Rank Ridge Regression) is proposed to fuse audios for voice based disease detection. First, the model couples the regression losses from two audios together to jointly learn a transformation matrix for each audio. Secondly, the conventional zero-one regression targets are relaxed by the ε-dragging technique so that the margins between different classes are enlarged. Third, low-rank constraint is imposed to exploit the correlation structure among different classes. The proposed algorithm not only enables to consider multiple audios, but also adjusts the weight of each audio adaptively. Due to the design of losses coupling, ε-dragging technique, and low-rank constraint, high performance is achieved. Experiments conducted on two disease detection tasks, each with six types of fusion, show that our fusion approach outperforms the case of using a single audio and another two fusion methods. Finally, key factors in JOLL4R are analyzed.

Keywords Joint learning · Ridge regression · Low-rank regression · ε-dragging technique · Voice based pathology detection

6.1 Introduction

Voice analysis is helpful to detect diseases, such as Parkinson's disease (PD) (Tsanas et al. 2012), Alzheimer's disease (Lopez-de Ipina et al. 2013), vocal cord paralysis (Saudi et al. 2012), and vocal cord nodule (Oguz et al. 2007; Maciel et al. 2007). In Tsanas et al. (2010), it was shown that voice analysis could even be used to predict the severity of PD. Compared with advanced diagnostic tools like laryngoscope and endoscope, voice analysis is non-invasive, painless, and convenient. The two most frequently adopted vocal tests are running speech and sustained vowels. For running speech, subjects are instructed to speak a pre-devised sentence containing representative linguistic units (Orozco-Arroyave et al. 2016). In terms of sustained vowels,

© Springer Nature Singapore Pte Ltd. 2020
D. Zhang, K. Wu, *Pathological Voice Analysis*,
https://doi.org/10.1007/978-981-32-9196-6_6

patients are asked to pronounce a vowel and sustain it as long as possible (Godino-Llorente et al. 2006). Since running speech is often coupled with confounding effects, most studies use a single vowel of normal pitch for analysis.

Voice based disease detection is a typical pattern recognition problem, in which discriminative features are designed to classify healthy and pathological voice (Maciel et al. 2007; Arias-Londono et al. 2010). Features proposed in the past literature can generally be categorized into three classes. First of all, there are features quantifying the periodicity extent since the vibration of vocal folds for pathological voice tends to deviate from periodicity. The two most representative features in this class are jitter and shimmer, which describe the perturbations of the fundamental frequency and amplitude over periods, respectively (Ludlow et al. 1987). Other features include GQ (glottal quotient) (Tsanas 2012), RPDE (recurrence period density entropy) (Little et al. 2007), and PPE (pitch period entropy) (Little et al. 2009). Features in the second group assess the noise extent in voice caused by incomplete glottal closures. HNR (harmonics to noise ratio), NHR (noise to harmonics ratio) (Yumoto et al. 1982), and DFA (detrended fluctuation analysis) (Little et al. 2007) are some of the classic features in this class. In the third category, features devised for speech and speaker recognition are adopted, such as MFCC (Mel-frequency cepstral coefficients) (Arias-Londono et al. 2010), LPC (linear prediction coefficients), and LPCC (linear prediction cepstral coefficients). Study in Mekyska et al. (2016) even indicated that features like LPC, LPCC, and MFCC outperformed conventional ones for PD detection.

Despite these proposed methods, we are motivated to investigate voice based disease detection through joint learning due to the following reasons. Firstly, considering different audios together is beneficial. Most existing methods use a single audio for disease detection, in which the sustained vowel /a/ produced with normal pitch is the dominant one. However, when a certain sample may not be accurately classified with features from one audio, it may be detected correctly if another audio is utilized. In addition, sometimes a patient is difficult to be detected with neither of the collected audios, whereas a combination of them may result in an accurate diagnosis. Therefore, it is meaningful to detect disease by fusing complementary information from different audios. Secondly, more effective fusion is needed. In the previous literature, there are three levels of fusion: (1) audio-level fusion concatenates different audios into a single recording (Maryn et al. 2010; Martinez et al. 2012a); (2) feature-level fusion concatenates feature vectors extracted from different audios into a single vector for classification (Vaiciukynas et al. 2014); (3) decision-level fusion, which is mostly used, combines the scores (or classification results) coming from different audios to obtain a higher accuracy (Vaiciukynas et al. 2014, 2016; Martinez et al. 2012a, b). While the first two types of fusion are quite simple, it may not be effective since the discriminative ability differences among different audios are ignored. Even though the decision-level fusion may show better performance than the first two (Vaiciukynas et al. 2014; Martinez et al. 2012a), it is time-consuming since it needs to train multiple classifiers. Therefore, it is necessary to explore a new type of fusion for voice based disease detection. With the above reasons taken into consideration, we aim to propose a voice fusion scheme, which is not only effective, but also requires less running time.

In this chapter, we propose a novel fusion model JOLL4R (JOint Learning based on Label Relaxed low-Rank Ridge Regression). Particularly, the proposed method couples the regression losses of two audios together to jointly learn a discriminative and compact transformation matrix for each audio. The label matrix is generated by relaxing the traditional binary regression targets to increase flexibility and to enlarge the margins between different classes. In addition, low-rank constraint and Tikhonov regularization terms are used to uncover the correlation structures between classes and to reduce the variance of the model, respectively. Finally, the performance of our model is assessed on different databases (each with six types of fusion) and key factors in the model are discussed in detail.

The rest of this chapter is organized as follows. Section 6.2 briefly presents related works. Details of our proposed joint learning algorithm are shown in Sect. 6.3. Sections 6.4 and 6.5 give experimental results and discussions, respectively. In Sect. 6.6, we conclude the chapter and present the future work.

6.2   Related Works

6.2.1   Notation

Matrices and column vectors in this chapter are denoted by bold uppercase letters and bold lower letters, respectively. A^T denotes the transposed matrix of A and I is an identity matrix. $\|A\|_F^2 = tr(A^T A) = tr(AA^T)$ stands for the squares of the Frobenius norm of matrix A, in which $tr(\cdot)$ is the trace operator. The nuclear norm of matrix A is represented by $\|A\|_*$.

6.2.2   Ridge Regression

Least square regression (LSR) is a fundamental technique in statistical analysis that is widely used in the field of pattern recognition. Not only is it mathematically tractable and computationally efficient, LSR is also effective for data analysis.

Given n training samples $\{x_1, x_2, \ldots, x_n\}$, we denote the data matrix as $X = \{x_1, x_2, \ldots, x_n\} \in R^{d \times n}$, where each column represents a sample and each row is a feature. The corresponding label matrix is denoted as $Y = \{y_1, y_2, \ldots, y_n\}^T \in R^{n \times c}$, where c is the number of classes. The purpose of LSR is to learn a projection matrix $W \in R^{d \times c}$ such that the projected feature matrix $X^T W$ can approximate the target matrix Y by minimizing the following objective function:

$$\min_{\mathbf{W}} \left\| \mathbf{X}^{\mathrm{T}}\mathbf{W} - \mathbf{Y} \right\|_F^2. \tag{6.1}$$

In the standard LSR, y_i in the label matrix Y is generally a zero-one vector, in which its kth entry is one and all the other are zero if x_i belongs to the kth class ($i = 1$, 2, ..., n and $k = 1$, 2, ..., c). As proved in (Hoerl and Kennard 1970), ridge regression, whose objective function is to add a Tikhonov regularization term to that of LSR, can achieve better performance since the regularization term helps to reduce the variance of the model by shrinking the coefficients in W. The model of ridge regression is formulated as:

$$\min_{\mathbf{W}} \left\| \mathbf{X}^{\mathrm{T}}\mathbf{W} - \mathbf{Y} \right\|_F^2 + \lambda_1 \|\mathbf{W}\|_F^2, \tag{6.2}$$

where λ_1 is the regularization parameter. Ridge regression has shown its effectiveness in many fields, such as subspace clustering (Peng et al. 2017), face recognition (Shin et al. 2007), and image denoising (Trinh et al. 2011). For more detailed analysis and extensions about ridge regression, readers may refer to the following works (Hoerl and Kennard 1970; Lai et al. 2018, 2019).

6.2.3 Low-Rank Ridge Regression

To explore and utilize the hidden correlation structure between classes, the Low-Rank Linear Regression (LRLR) model was proposed (Cai et al. 2013). Different from the Frobenius norm based regularization in ridge regression, a nuclear norm regularization is imposed on the objective function, as formulated below.

$$\min_{\mathbf{W}} \left\| \mathbf{X}^{\mathrm{T}}\mathbf{W} - \mathbf{Y} \right\|_F^2 + \lambda_2 \|\mathbf{W}\|_*, \tag{6.3}$$

where λ_2 is the low-rank regularization parameter. The last term in Eq. (6.3) helps to learn a compact low-rank projection matrix W so that the low-rank structures between classes can be discovered and utilized (Wong et al. 2017). In Cai et al. (2013), it was proved that the LRLR model was equivalent to linear regression in the linear discriminant analysis subspace.

The Frobenius and nuclear norm of the projection matrix W in Eqs. (6.2) and (6.3) are in fact the l_2-norm and l_1-norm of the singular values of W, respectively (Zhang et al. 2017). As discussed (Grave et al. 2011; Wright et al. 2009; Feng and Zhou 2016; Zou and Hastie 2005; Lai et al. 2016; Cao et al. 2018), it is advisable to combine the benefits of l_2-norm and l_1-norm together for improvements. Hence, these two terms were added to LSR (Cai et al. 2013), forming the Low-Rank Ridge Regression (LRRR) as presented below, so that a compact and discriminative projection W could be learned.

$$\min_{\mathbf{W}} \left\|\mathbf{X}^{\mathrm{T}}\mathbf{W} - \mathbf{Y}\right\|_F^2 + \lambda_1 \|\mathbf{W}\|_F^2 + \lambda_2 \|\mathbf{W}\|_* \tag{6.4}$$

Comparing with LSR, elastic-net regularization (i.e., the l_2-norm and l_1-norm regularization) of singular values are added in the objective function of LRRR as shown in Eq. (6.4). As discussed (Zhang et al. 2017), the l_2-norm regularization helps to shrink a variable towards zero but tends to keep all components in the variable. Hence, predictors obtained by using l_2-norm regularization only may contain redundant information. In contrast, l_1-norm regularization is useful to generate sparse result so that principal information can be selected. Nevertheless, adopting l_1-norm regularization only can result in sub-optimal results since it generally selects only one component for a group of highly correlated variables. In LRRR, the l_2-norm and l_1-norm regularization are combined so that grouped principal components can be selected and redundancies in data can be reduced simultaneously.

6.2.4 ε-Dragging Technique

The zero-one entries in the label matrix limit the power of LSR for data classification, especially for multi-class classification tasks, since the zero-one targets are too rigid to learn (Zhang et al. 2015). To make LSR more appropriate for classification, some variants of LSR revise the loss function of LSR, such as least squares support vector machine (Van Gestel et al. 2002; Brabanter et al. 2012) and discriminatively regularized LSR (Xue et al. 2009). Other studies, however, try to transform the regression targets in LSR so that the targets are less rigid and the margins between different classes are as large as possible (Zhang et al. 2015; Xiang et al. 2012). In Zhang et al. (2015), it was put forward to learn the regression targets and a framework of retargeted least squares for multi-class classification was presented. In Xiang et al. (2012), Xiang et al. proposed a framework of discriminative least square regression (DLSR) for classification by introducing the ε-dragging technique to modify the regression targets. In Fang et al. (2018), Fang et al. adopted the same ε-dragging technique and proposed a regularized label relaxation model for classification.

For each label vector y_i from the kth class, the ε-dragging technique is to drag the binary entries far away along two opposite directions so that the kth entry in y_i "1" becomes "$1 + \epsilon_{i1}$" and other entries "0"s are changed to "$-\epsilon_{i0}^j$," where "ϵ_{i1}" and "ϵ_{i0}^j" are positive slack variables ($i \in \{1, \cdots, n\}, j \in \{1, \cdots, c, j \neq k\}$). In this way, the ε-dragging relaxes the strict binary regression target matrix to soft extent to gain more flexibility to fit the data. Meanwhile, it also enlarges the distance between any two data points from different classes, which is generally desired for classification tasks. For more details of ε-dragging, please refer to the paper (Xiang et al. 2012).

The label relaxed LSR model, which is to introduce the ε-dragging into LSR, can be denoted as

$$\min_{\mathbf{W}} \left\| \mathbf{X}^{\mathsf{T}}\mathbf{W} - \widehat{\mathbf{Y}} \right\|_F^2, \tag{6.5}$$

where $\widehat{\mathbf{Y}}$ is the relaxed regression target matrix. For optimization, the relaxed matrix is constructed by $\widehat{\mathbf{Y}} = \mathbf{Y} + \mathbf{E} \odot \mathbf{M}$, where E is a devised constant matrix and M is a nonnegative matrix to be learned. The definition of E is

$$E_{ij} = \begin{cases} +1 & \text{if } Y_{ij} = 1 \\ -1 & \text{if } Y_{ij} = 0 \end{cases} \tag{6.6}$$

Therefore, Eq. (6.5) is rewritten as follows. Note that each entry of M is nonnegative so that the dragging can be conducted with the direction decided in matrix E.

$$\min_{\mathbf{W},\mathbf{M}} \left\| \mathbf{X}^{\mathsf{T}}\mathbf{W} - \left(\mathbf{Y} + \mathbf{E} \odot \mathbf{M} \right) \right\|_F^2 \quad \text{s.t.} \quad \mathbf{M} \geqslant \mathbf{0} \tag{6.7}$$

6.3   Proposed Method

6.3.1   Joint Learning with Label Relaxed Low-Rank Ridge Regression (JOLL4R)

Applying the ε-dragging technique to the LRRR model, we can formulate an improved model.

$$\min_{\mathbf{W},\mathbf{M}} \left\| \mathbf{X}^{\mathsf{T}}\mathbf{W} - \left(\mathbf{Y} + \mathbf{E} \odot \mathbf{M} \right) \right\|_F^2 + \lambda_1 \|\mathbf{W}\|_F^2 + \lambda_2 \|\mathbf{W}\|_* \quad \text{s.t.} \quad \mathbf{M} \geqslant \mathbf{0}. \tag{6.8}$$

While voice based pathology detection is traditionally realized by analyzing a single voice signal, we attempt to enhance the performance with two different voice signals. Notice that the model can be extended to the fusion of more voice signals (≥ 3), as discussed in Sect. 6.5.3. Denote the feature matrices from two voice signals as X_1 and X_2, and the corresponding transformation matrices as W_1 and W_2, respectively. Then the proposed JOint Learning based on Label Relaxed low-Rank Ridge Regression (JOLL4R) is formulated as

$$\min_{\mathbf{W_1},\mathbf{W_2},\mathbf{M}} \left\| \frac{1}{2}\mathbf{X_1}^\mathsf{T}\mathbf{W_1} + \frac{1}{2}\mathbf{X_2}^\mathsf{T}\mathbf{W_2} - \left(\mathbf{Y} + \mathbf{E}\bigodot\mathbf{M}\right) \right\|_F^2 + \lambda_{11}\|\mathbf{W_1}\|_F^2 + \lambda_{12}\|\mathbf{W_1}\|_*$$
$$+\lambda_{21}\|\mathbf{W_2}\|_F^2 + \lambda_{22}\|\mathbf{W_2}\|_* \quad \text{s.t.} \quad \mathbf{M} \geqslant \mathbf{0},$$

$$(6.9)$$

where the first term represents the least square loss and the last four are regularization terms. λ_{11}, λ_{12}, λ_{21}, and λ_{22} are the corresponding regularization parameters to be optimized experimentally. While it seems that the weights for two voices in the first term are the same (both 0.5), we argue that the contributions of different signals can be reflected with the energies of the learned projections. It is easy to see that the following equation holds:

$$\frac{1}{2}\mathbf{X_1}^\mathsf{T}\mathbf{W_1} + \frac{1}{2}\mathbf{X_2}^\mathsf{T}\mathbf{W_2} = \frac{\|\mathbf{W_1}\|_F^2}{2} \times \frac{\mathbf{X_1}^\mathsf{T}\mathbf{W_1}}{\|\mathbf{W_1}\|_F^2} + \frac{\|\mathbf{W_2}\|_F^2}{2} \times \frac{\mathbf{X_2}^\mathsf{T}\mathbf{W_2}}{\|\mathbf{W_2}\|_F^2}.$$

Evidently, a larger energy of the learned projection matrix indicates a higher weight on this voice. Instead of expressing losses as $\frac{1}{2}\|\mathbf{X_1}^\mathsf{T}\mathbf{W_1} - (\mathbf{Y} + \mathbf{E}\bigodot\mathbf{M})\|_F^2 + \frac{1}{2}\|\mathbf{X_2}^\mathsf{T}\mathbf{W_2} - (\mathbf{Y} + \mathbf{E}\bigodot\mathbf{M})\|_F^2$ the first term in Eq. (6.9) couples the losses from two audios together by using a single Frobenius norm, which makes the estimating of W_1 dependent on that of W_2 and vice versa. In this way, W_1 and W_2 cooperate with each other to regress the target label jointly. When the model in Eq. (6.9) is used on a single voice, it will be degenerated to the method in Zhang et al. (2017) for image classification, in which the model was referred to as DENLR (Discriminative Elastic-Net regularized Linear Regression).

6.3.2 Algorithm to Solve JOLL4R

In this section, we tackle the problem in Eq. (6.9) by proposing an efficient algorithm via the augmented Lagrangian method (ALM), in which Eq. (6.9) has a closed-form solution in each iteration. First of all, an equation regarding the nuclear norm regularization in Eq. (6.9) holds (Mazumder et al. 2010).

$$\|\mathbf{W}\|_* = \min_{\mathbf{W=AB}} \frac{1}{2}\left(\|\mathbf{A}\|_F^2 + \|\mathbf{B}\|_F^2\right), \quad (6.10)$$

where $A \in R^{d \times r}$, $B \in R^{r \times c}$, and $r < \min(d,c)$. Applying Eq. (6.10) to our model, Eq. (6.9) can be rewritten as

$$\min_{W_1, W_2, M, A_1, B_1, A_2, B_2} \left\| \frac{1}{2} X_1{}^T W_1 + \frac{1}{2} X_2{}^T W_2 - \left(Y + E \bigodot M \right) \right\|_F^2$$

$$+ \lambda_{11} \| W_1 \|_F^2 + \frac{\lambda_{12}}{2} \left(\| A_1 \|_F^2 + \| B_1 \|_F^2 \right) + \frac{\lambda_{22}}{2} \left(\| A_2 \|_F^2 + \| B_2 \|_F^2 \right)$$

$$+ \lambda_{21} \| W_2 \|_F^2 \quad \text{s.t.} \quad M \geqslant 0,$$

$$W_1 = A_1 B_1, W_2 = A_2 B_2. \tag{6.11}$$

We use the augmented Lagrangian function to replace Eq. (6.11)

$$L(W_1, W_2, M, A_1, B_1, A_2, B_2) = \left\| \frac{1}{2} \left(X_1{}^T W_1 + X_2{}^T W_2 \right) - \left(Y + E \bigodot M \right) \right\|_F^2$$

$$+ \lambda_{11} \| W_1 \|_F^2 + \langle C_1, W_1 - A_1 B_1 \rangle + \frac{\mu_1}{2} \| W_1 - A_1 B_1 \|_F^2$$

$$+ \lambda_{21} \| W_2 \|_F^2 + \langle C_2, W_2 - A_2 B_2 \rangle + \frac{\mu_2}{2} \| W_2 - A_2 B_2 \|_F^2$$

$$+ \frac{\lambda_{12}}{2} \left(\| A_1 \|_F^2 + \| B_1 \|_F^2 \right) + \frac{\lambda_{22}}{2} \left(\| A_2 \|_F^2 + \| B_2 \|_F^2 \right) \tag{6.12}$$

where $\langle S, T \rangle = tr(S^T T)$, C_1 and C_2 are Lagrange multipliers, and μ_1 and μ_2 are the penalty parameters. Then Eq. (6.12) can be solved alternatively with the following steps.

Step 1 Fix other variables, minimize the function over A_1 (A_2). First, update A_1 by solving the following problem, where terms irrelevant to A_1 are discarded:

$$A_1^+ = \arg \min_{A_1} \frac{\lambda_{12}}{2} \| A_1 \|_F^2 + \langle C_1, W_1 - A_1 B_1 \rangle + \frac{\mu_1}{2} \| W_1 - A_1 B_1 \|_F^2$$

$$= \arg \min_{A_1} \frac{\lambda_{12}}{2} \| A_1 \|_F^2 + \frac{\mu_1}{2} \left\| W_1 - A_1 B_1 + \frac{C_1}{\mu_1} \right\|_F^2. \tag{6.13}$$

Clearly, Problem (6.13) is a regularized least square problem with the solution presented below.

$$A_1^+ = (C_1 + \mu_1 W_1) B_1{}^T \left(\lambda_{12} I + \mu_1 B_1 B_1{}^T \right)^{-1}. \tag{6.14}$$

Due to the symmetry between A_1 and A_2, we can derive the solution to update A_2, as in Eq. (6.15).

$$A_2^+ = (C_2 + \mu_2 W_2) B_2{}^T \left(\lambda_{22} I + \mu_2 B_2 B_2{}^T \right)^{-1}. \tag{6.15}$$

Step 2 Update B_1 (B_2) after keeping other variables fixed. The problem to be solved is

$$\begin{aligned}
\mathbf{B_1^+} &= \arg\min_{\mathbf{B_1}} \frac{\lambda_{12}}{2} \|\mathbf{B_1}\|_F^2 + \langle \mathbf{C_1}, \mathbf{W_1} - \mathbf{A_1B_1} \rangle + \frac{\mu_1}{2} \|\mathbf{W_1} - \mathbf{A_1B_1}\|_F^2 \\
&= \arg\min_{\mathbf{B_1}} \frac{\lambda_{12}}{2} \|\mathbf{B_1}\|_F^2 + \frac{\mu_1}{2} \left\| \mathbf{W_1} - \mathbf{A_1B_1} + \frac{\mathbf{C_1}}{\mu_1} \right\|_F^2.
\end{aligned}$$

(6.16)

It is easy to find that the solution to Problem (6.16) is

$$\mathbf{B_1^+} = \left(\lambda_{12}\mathbf{I} + \mu_1 \mathbf{A_1}^T \mathbf{A_1} \right)^{-1} \mathbf{A_1}^T (\mathbf{C_1} + \mu_1 \mathbf{W_1}).$$

(6.17)

Similar to B_1, B_2 can be updated by

$$\mathbf{B_2^+} = \left(\lambda_{22}\mathbf{I} + \mu_2 \mathbf{A_2}^T \mathbf{A_2} \right)^{-1} \mathbf{A_2}^T (\mathbf{C_2} + \mu_2 \mathbf{W_2}).$$

(6.18)

Step 3 Update the transformation matrix W_1 (W_2). When other variables are fixed, we have the following optimization problem for W_1:

$$\begin{aligned}
\mathbf{W_1^+} &= \arg\min_{\mathbf{W_1}} \left\| \frac{1}{2} (\mathbf{X_1}^T \mathbf{W_1} + \mathbf{X_2}^T \mathbf{W_2}) - \left(\mathbf{Y} + \mathbf{E} \bigodot \mathbf{M} \right) \right\|_F^2 + \lambda_{11} \|\mathbf{W_1}\|_F^2 \\
&\quad + \langle \mathbf{C_1}, \mathbf{W_1} - \mathbf{A_1B_1} \rangle + \frac{\mu_1}{2} \|\mathbf{W_1} - \mathbf{A_1B_1}\|_F^2 \\
&= \arg\min_{\mathbf{W_1}} \left\| \frac{1}{2} (\mathbf{X_1}^T \mathbf{W_1} + \mathbf{X_2}^T \mathbf{W_2}) \right. \\
&\quad - \left. \left(\mathbf{Y} + \mathbf{E} \bigodot \mathbf{M} \right) \right\|_F^2 + \lambda_{11} \|\mathbf{W_1}\|_F^2 \\
&\quad + \frac{\mu_1}{2} \left\| \mathbf{W_1} - \mathbf{A_1B_1} + \frac{\mathbf{C_1}}{\mu_1} \right\|_F^2
\end{aligned}$$

(6.19)

By setting derivative of Problem (6.19) with respect to W_1 to zero, the optimal solution can be calculated by

$$\mathbf{W_1^+} = \left(\frac{1}{2} \mathbf{X_1}\mathbf{X_1}^T + 2\lambda_{11}\mathbf{I} + \mu_1\mathbf{I} \right)^{-1} \left(\mathbf{X_1P} - \frac{1}{2} \mathbf{X_1}\mathbf{X_2}^T \mathbf{W_2} + \mu_1 \mathbf{A_1B_1} - \mathbf{C_1} \right),$$

(6.20)

where $\mathbf{P} = \mathbf{Y} + \mathbf{E} \odot \mathbf{M}$. Again, the symmetry between W_1 and W_2 helps us to derive the solution of W_2.

$$\mathbf{W}_2^+ = \left(\frac{1}{2}\mathbf{X}_2\mathbf{X}_2^\mathrm{T} + 2\lambda_{21}\mathbf{I} + \mu_2\mathbf{I}\right)^{-1}\left(\mathbf{X}_2\mathbf{P} - \frac{1}{2}\mathbf{X}_2\mathbf{X}_1^\mathrm{T}\mathbf{W}_1 + \mu_1\mathbf{A}_2\mathbf{B}_2 - \mathbf{C}_2\right)$$

$$\tag{6.21}$$

Step 4 To update M, the following problem is to be solved:

$$\mathbf{M}^+ = \arg\min_{\mathbf{M}} \left\| \frac{1}{2}\left(\mathbf{X}_1^\mathrm{T}\mathbf{W}_1 + \mathbf{X}_2^\mathrm{T}\mathbf{W}_2\right) - \left(\mathbf{Y} + \mathbf{E}\bigodot\mathbf{M}\right) \right\|_F^2 \quad \text{s.t.} \ \ \mathbf{M} \geqslant \mathbf{0}. \ \ (6.22)$$

According to the work in Xiang et al. (2012), the solution to Problem (6.22) is

$$\mathbf{M}^+ = \max\left(\left(\frac{1}{2}\left(\mathbf{X}_1^\mathrm{T}\mathbf{W}_1 + \mathbf{X}_2^\mathrm{T}\mathbf{W}_2\right) - \mathbf{Y}\right)\bigodot\mathbf{E}, \mathbf{0}\right).$$

$$\tag{6.23}$$

We continue to alternately solve for A_1, A_2, B_1, B_2, W_1, W_2, and M by Eqs. (6.14), (6.15), (6.17), (6.18), (6.20), (6.21), and (6.23) until a maximum number of iterations is reached or a predefined threshold is reached.

Step 5 The Lagrange multipliers C_1 and C_2 are updated by Eqs. (6.24) and (6.25), respectively.

$$\mathbf{C}_1 = \mathbf{C}_1 + \mu_1(\mathbf{W}_1 - \mathbf{A}_1\mathbf{B}_1). \tag{6.24}$$

$$\mathbf{C}_2 = \mathbf{C}_2 + \mu_2(\mathbf{W}_2 - \mathbf{A}_2\mathbf{B}_2).. \tag{6.25}$$

The algorithm of JOLL4R is described in Algorithm 6.1.

6.3.3 Classification

After solving JOLL4R, the two projection matrices W_1 and W_2 are obtained, with which we utilize to make linear transformations for the feature matrices of both training and test samples. Then the simple nearest neighbor (1-NN) classifier follows to perform the final classification. Besides, as presented in Sect. 6.4.1, the sample size for our binary classification tasks is imbalanced, which leads to the class imbalance issue. Here, the ADAptive SYNthetic sampling (ADASYN) (He et al. 2008) is utilized to generate synthetic samples of the minority class.

Algorithm 6.1 Optimization of JOLL4R

Input: Feature matrices: X_1, X_2; Label matrix: Y; Constant Matrix: E;
   Initialization: Initialize $W_1 \in R^{d \times c}$, $W_2 \in R^{d \times c}$, $A_1 \in R^{d \times r}$, $A_2 \in R^{d \times r}$, $B_1 \in Rr \times c$, $B_2 \in Rr \times c$, $C_1 \in Rd \times c$, and $C_2 \in Rd \times c$ randomly, $M = 0$, $\lambda_{11} > 0$, $\lambda_{12} > 0$, $\lambda_{21} > 0$, $\lambda_{22} > 0$, $\mu_1 > 0$, $\mu_2 > 0$.

1. **while** not converged **do**
2. **while** not converged **do**
3. **Step 1** Update A_1 and A_2 according to Eqs. (6.14) and (6.15), respectively.
4. **Step 2** Update B_1 and B_2 according to Eqs. (6.17) and (6.18), respectively.
5. **Step 3** Update W_1 and W_2 according to Eqs. (6.20) and (6.21), respectively.
6. **Step 4** Update M according to Eq. (6.23).
7. **end while**
8. **Step 5** Update C_1 and C_2 according to Eqs. (6.24) and (6.25), respectively.
9. **end while**

   Output: The Optimal Projection Matrices: W_1 and W_2.
   with which to compensate for the skewed distribution so that the distribution of the resulting dataset is more balanced. Note that the synthetic samples are used for training only. The effect of ADASYN is discussed experimentally in Sect. 6.4.4. For clarity, we summarize the whole classification procedures in Algorithm 6.2.

Algorithm 6.2 Optimization of JOLL4R

Input: Training feature sets: X_{tr1} and X_{tr2}; Label matrix for training samples: Y_{tr}; Test feature sets: X_{te1} and X_{te2};
   Step 1 Adopt ADASYN on X_{tr1} (and X_{tr2}) to generate synthetic samples of the minority class, denoted as X_{sy1} (and X_{sy2}).
   Step 2 Add the synthetic samples X_{sy1} (and X_{sy2}) to the original training feature X_{tr1} (and X_{tr2}) to obtain a balanced dataset X_{tr1} (and X_{tr2})
   Step 3 Employ X_{tr1} and X_{tr2} as the input to Algorithm 6.1 to obtain the two projection matrices W_1 and W_2.
   Step 4 Transform X_{tr1} and X_{tr2} linearly with the projection matrices W_1 and W_2, respectively, to form the new training set: $X_{trtr}^{F} = \frac{1}{2} X_{tr1}^{T} W_1 + \frac{1}{2} X_{tr2}^{T} W_2$.
   Similarly, the fused test set can be obtained by: $X_{te}^{F} = \frac{1}{2} X_{te1}^{T} W_1 + \frac{1}{2} X_{te2}^{T} W_2$.
   Step 5 Predict the labels Y_{te} for X_{te}^{F} using the nearest neighbor (1-NN) classifier.
   Output: The Predicted Label Matrix Y_{te} for test samples.

6.4 Experimental Results

6.4.1 Dataset and Experimental Setup

The freely available database Saarbruecken Voice Database (SVD) is used (Barry and Putzer) in our experiments, in which recordings for each speaker include vowels /a/, /i/, and /u/ produced at normal, low, high, and low-high-low pitch, together with a sentence. This database is quite new, on which few studies have been conducted (Al-nasheri et al. 2017; Muhammad et al. 2017). In this chapter, we use the vowel /a/ produced at any two of the four different pitch types for fusion. More details about the experimental setting and results are presented in literature (Wu et al. 2019).

In this section, we conduct two classification tasks: (1) healthy versus cordectomy and (2) healthy versus frontolateral resection. Examples of voice signals from healthy subject and patient are given in Fig. 6.1, and periods are divided by red lines. Evidently, there are large extents of dissimilarities among the eight periods, indicating irregularity of vocal folds or vocal tracts for this patient.

Considering the imbalance issue, we adopt similar metrics used in Chap. 5: sensitivity (*Sen*), specificity (*Spe*), and the geometric mean (*Gmean*), which is seen as the main metric in our class imbalanced tasks. Note that positive and negative classes refer to patients with cordectomy (frontolateral resection) and healthy subjects, respectively.

The perturbation of fundamental frequency and amplitude of voice over periods increases when the vocal cords of patients cannot function normally. Hence, jitter and shimmer, both of which have 22 variants, are used as features in our work and

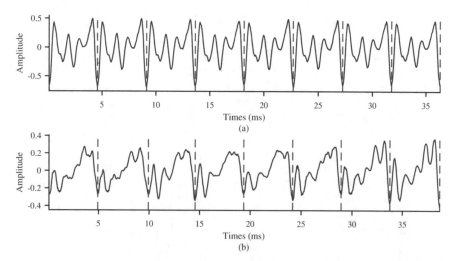

Fig. 6.1 (color online) Waveform segment from two individuals. The audio used is the vowel /a/ produced with a normal pitch. (**a**) segment from a healthy subject. (**b**) voice segment from a patient with frontolateral resection. In each plot, the dotted red vertical lines are added to separate the segment into eight periods approximately

presented in detail in Tsanas et al. (2012). Then principal component analysis (PCA) follows to reduce the high correlation, in which the reduced dimension is estimated by the maximum likelihood method (Levina and Bickel 2005). In the assessment of JOLL4R, four other methods are added for comparison. The first two are the results of the degenerated model DENLR (Zhang et al. 2017) used on each of the two audio signals. The third one is to apply the features averaged over the two audio signals on DENLR, which is denoted as DENLR-M. Finally, the naive way of fusion that concatenates features extracted from two audios, is added, in which the nearest neighbor (1-NN) classifier is used for classification (denoted by CONC). Each result is represented by "mean $\pm$ standard deviation %."

6.4.2 The Detection of Patients with Cordectomy

Table 6.1 shows the performance of five methods in detecting patients with cordectomy. The symbol of "n-l" in this table represents that the two audios for fusion are the vowels produced at normal and low pitch. Audios participating in other fusion can be known similarly from the symbols in first column. Overall, the proposed method JOLL4R always gives the highest *Gmean* for any pair of fusion. The corresponding deviations are either the lowest or comparable to the lowest. In addition, JOLL4R also achieves the highest *Sen* for all six pairs of fusion.

6.4.3 The Detection of Patients with Frontolateral Resection

The results of five methods in detecting patients with frontolateral resection are shown in Table 6.2. As before, *Gmean* is the main metric in comparison. In each pair of fusion, JOLL4R outperforms DENLR used on participating audios separately. Comparing with DENLR-M, JOLL4R achieves higher *Gmean* in five out of six pairs. Besides, a statistical significance test was conducted to show the advantages of JOLL4R over DENLR-M more obviously, with the *p*-values presented in Table 6.3. Combining Tables 6.2 and 6.3, it can be seen that JOLL4R outperforms DENLR-M in most cases. Finally, as in detecting cordectomy, JOLL4R is superior to the CONC method in all six pairs of fusion.

6.4.4 Ablation Study

In this part, we experimentally explore the impact of each key component in JOLL4R, such as the low-rank constraint, ε-dragging technique, and ADASYN strategy that deals with the class imbalance problem.

Table 6.1 The performance of different models in cordectomy detection

Audios	Models	Gmean (%)	Sen (%)	Spe (%)
n-l	DENLR(n)	81.23 ± 7.55	79.05 ± 14.52	84.36 ± 3.91
	DENLR(l)	71.12 ± 8.83	66.35 ± 16.36	77.73 ± 4.50
	DENLR-M	80.83 ± 6.80	78.72 ± 13.78	83.86 ± 3.98
	CONT	76.27 ± 9.97	63.60 ± 16.03	**93.14 ± 2.42**
	JOLL4R	**82.48 ± 6.85**	**80.35 ± 13.62**	85.54 ± 3.93
n-h	DENLR(n)	81.46 ± 7.23	79.45 ± 14.01	84.38 ± 3.94
	DENLR(h)	78.59 ± 8.96	73.60 ±16.22	85.24 ± 4.02
	DENLR-M	79.39 ± 7.52	78.63 ± 14.69	81.14 ± 4.02
	CONT	79.18 ± 9.55	67.50 ± 15.37	**94.31 ± 2.15**
	JOLL4R	**84.26 ± 6.49**	**82.88 ± 13.25**	86.42 ± 3.72
n-lhl	DENLR(n)	81.45 ± 7.21	79.57 ± 14.00	84.22 ± 3.65
	DENLR(lhl)	78.24 ± 7.73	73.45 ± 14.64	84.44 ± 4.15
	DENLR-M	75.30 ± 8.07	72.20 ± 15.58	79.78 ± 4.29
	CONT	80.14 ± 9.07	68.58 ± 15.05	**94.96 ± 2.09**
	JOLL4R	**85.86 ± 6.45**	**83.55 ± 12.88**	88.92 ± 3.35
l-h	DENLR(l)	70.89 ± 9.09	66.07 ± 16.43	77.54 ± 4.26
	DENLR(h)	78.77 ± 8.77	73.90 ± 16.35	85.32 ± 4.10
	DENLR-M	79.41 ± 7.06	**77.63 ± 14.08**	82.15 ± 4.06
	CONT	73.21 ± 10.70	59.08 ± 16.67	**92.83 ± 2.42**
	JOLL4R	**80.01 ± 7.22**	76.78 ± 14.21	84.39 ± 4.18
l-lhl	DENLR(l)	70.94 ± 8.54	66.05 ± 15.60	77.53 ± 4.11
	DENLR(lhl)	78.03 ± 7.54	73.40 ± 14.46	84.04 ± 4.10
	DENLR-M	76.45 ± 7.81	73.75 ± 15.13	80.36 ± 4.32
	CONT	71.21 ± 10.45	56.30 ± 15.70	**92.18 ± 2.55**
	JOLL4R	**79.81 ± 7.54**	**77.08 ± 14.63**	83.66 ± 4.08
h-lhl	DENLR(h)	79.52 ± 8.14	75.15 ± 15.22	85.25 ± 3.89
	DENLR(lhl)	77.59 ± 7.67	72.55 ± 14.62	84.11 ± 4.08
	DENLR-M	80.13 ± 7.45	77.15 ± 13.97	84.08 ± 3.85
	CONT	76.60 ± 9.84	62.9 ± 15.58	**94.91 ± 2.15**
	JOLL4R	**82.83 ± 6.71**	**80.47 ± 13.28**	86.06 ± 3.93

Bold values indicate better results

6.4.4.1 Parameters Sensitivity Analysis

In this section, the sensitivity of parameters λ_{11}, λ_{12}, λ_{21}, and λ_{22} in JOLL4R is analyzed. Results in the fusion of "n-lhl" (which shows the highest *Gmean*) in cordectomy detection are given. Figure 6.2 illustrates the *Gmean* versus the different values of parameters λ_{11} and λ_{21}, which control the energies of the learned projection W_1 and W_2, respectively. It can be noted that the optimal value of λ_{21} is larger than that of λ_{11}, suggesting that audio 1 (pitch "n") is more important than audio 2 (pitch "lhl") in the fusion. From Table 6.1, we indeed find out that DENLR used on audio

Table 6.2 Performance of different models in frontolateral resection detection

Audios	Models	Gmean (%)	Sen (%)	Spe (%)
n-l	DENLR(n)	93.14 ± 6.67	89.71 ± 12.48	97.25 ± 1.54
	DENLR(l)	83.97 ± 10.20	78.10 ± 18.06	91.81 ± 2.98
	DENLR-M	93.61 ± 5.42	91.79 ± 10.85	95.89 ± 2.11
	CONT	87.32 ± 9.31	78.89 ± 16.18	**97.78 ± 1.20**
	JOLL4R	**94.46 ± 5.94**	**91.88 ± 11.33**	97.55 ± 1.42
n-h	DENLR(n)	93.49 ± 6.97	90.37 ± 12.96	97.32 ± 1.52
	DENLR(h)	87.90 ± 8.21	83.79 ± 15.11	93.13 ± 2.31
	DENLR-M	92.46 ± 6.75	89.77 ± 12.74	95.81 ± 1.83
	CONT	87.67 ± 9.44	79.11 ± 16.19	**98.31 ± 1.11**
	JOLL4R	**94.57 ± 5.94**	**92.41 ± 11.39**	97.23 ± 1.52
n-lhl	DENLR(n)	92.92 ± 7.40	89.42 ± 13.77	97.25 ± 1.44
	DENLR(lhl)	88.11 ± 8.66	82.81 ± 15.81	94.82 ± 2.80
	DENLR-M	93.25 ± 5.48	**92.27 ± 11.3**	94.75 ± 2.72
	CONT	91.06 ± 8.03	85.07 ± 14.40	**98.26 ± 1.12**
	JOLL4R	**93.44 ± 5.73**	91.56 ± 11.56	95.87 ± 2.58
l-h	DENLR(l)	84.49 ± 9.33	78.85 ± 16.71	91.84 ± 2.99
	DENLR(h)	88.26 ± 7.64	84.50 ± 14.22	92.96 ± 2.31
	DENLR-M	89.55 ± 8.02	86.17 ± 14.91	93.94 ± 2.27
	CONT	84.54 ± 9.89	74.67 ± 16.65	**97.06 ± 1.55**
	JOLL4R	**90.14 ± 7.08**	**86.91 ± 13.44**	94.19 ± 2.27
l-lhl	DENLR(l)	84.48 ± 9.61	78.82 ± 16.93	91.85 ± 3.02
	DENLR(lhl)	87.68 ± 8.33	81.99 ± 15.52	94.78 ± 2.88
	DENLR-M	**91.64 ± 6.11**	**90.33 ± 12.15**	93.53 ± 2.72
	CONT	81.16 ± 11.44	69.51 ± 18.76	**96.74 ± 1.65**
	JOLL4R	89.97 ± 6.93	86.11 ± 13.32	94.70 ± 2.49
h-lhl	DENLR(h)	87.73 ± 8.22	83.51 ± 14.82	93.06 ± 2.38
	DENLR(lhl)	88.14 ± 8.60	82.97 ± 15.72	94.70 ± 2.89
	DENLR-M	90.87 ± 6.68	88.75 ± 13.06	93.70 ± 2.57
	CONT	84.26 ± 9.94	73.86 ± 16.81	**97.5 ± 1.36**
	JOLL4R	**91.60 ± 6.77**	**89.39 ± 13.39**	94.59 ± 3.02

Bold values indicate better results

Table 6.3 p-values between JOLL4R and DENLR-M

Audios	p-values	Audios	p-values
n-l	1.04×10^{-5}	l-h	2.44×10^{-32}
n-h	8.77×10^{-5}	l-lhl	7.92×10^{-29}
n-lhl	0.1256	h-lhl	3.71×10^{-19}

of pitch "n" achieves better performance than that on pitch "lhl." The above explanation holds true for other types of fusion.

Figure 6.3 illustrates the influence of parameters λ_{12} and λ_{22}, which are the regularization parameters imposed on the nuclear norm of projection matrices W_1 and W_2, respectively. It is evident that the highest *Gmean* is achieved when both λ_{12}

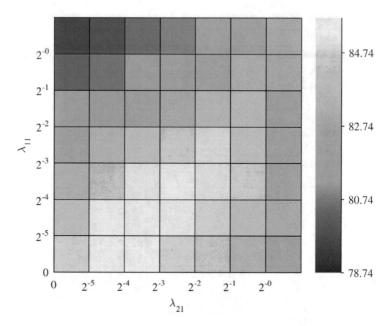

Fig. 6.2 (color online) *Gmean* versus different values of λ_{11} and λ_{21} for "n-lhl" fusion

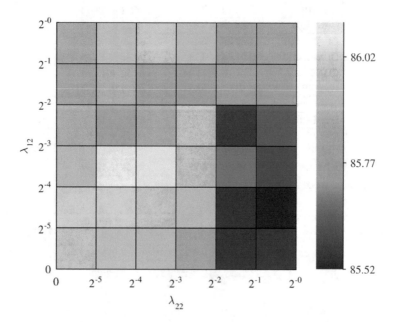

Fig. 6.3 (color online) *Gmean* versus different values of λ_{12} and λ_{22} for "n-lhl" fusion

Table 6.4 The performance with and without ε-dragging

ε-dragging	Gmean (%)	Sen (%)	Spe (%)
Yes	**85.51±6.11**	**83±12.43**	**88.76±3.52**
No	82.08±6.82	78.77±13.33	86.3±3.6

Bold values indicate better results

Table 6.5 The performance with and without ADASYN

ADASYN	Gmean (%)	Sen (%)	Spe (%)
Yes	**85.51 ± 6.61**	**83.03 ± 12.94**	88.77 ± 3.4
No	78.23 ± 10.64	63.68 ± 16.38	**97.93 ± 1.29**

Bold values indicate better results

and λ_{22} are nonzero. Therefore, the low-rank regularization is needed for superior performance.

6.4.4.2 The Effect of the ε-Dragging Technique

Table 6.4 displays the changes of performance when JOLL4R is deprived of the ε-dragging, in which the label matrix is replaced with the conventional zero-one entries. It can be found that *Gmean*, *Sen*, and *Spe* all drop when ε-dragging is removed. Comparing with the traditional binary label matrix, the regression target after adopting ε-dragging technique is more flexible and the margins between different classes are enlarged at the same time so that the learned projections W_1 and W_2 are more discriminative.

6.4.4.3 The Effect of ADASYN

The experimental results with and without ADASYN are shown in Table 6.5. When JOLL4R is used directly without ADASYN, most samples of interest (patients with cordectomy in this case) are classified as healthy. With ADASYN, *Gmean* increases significantly.

6.5 Discussions

6.5.1 Visualization of JOLL4R

In JOLL4R, two matrices W_1 and W_2 are learned, with which the two feature vectors (from the two audios of the same subject) are linearly transformed and then fused into a single vector. In this part, we visualize the features before and after the transformation to show the effectiveness of JOLL4R intuitively.

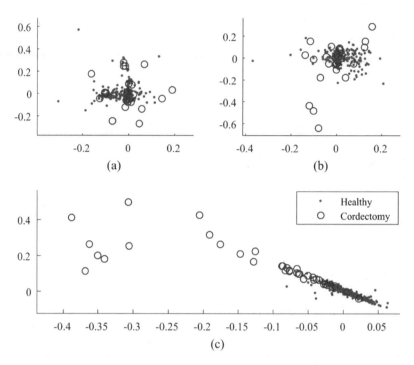

Fig. 6.4 (color online) The visualization of the original features (first two principal components) and the features generated by JOLL4R. (**a**) features of audio "n." (**b**) features of audio "lhl." (**c**) features transformed by JOLL4R

Table 6.6 Performance with different classifiers used for JOLL4R

Classifier	Gmean (%)	Sen (%)	Spe (%)
1-NN	85.77 ± 5.99	83.60 ± 11.99	88.60 ± 3.41
SVM	**87.86 ± 6.32**	**84.03 ± 12.08**	**92.43 ± 2.37**

Bold values indicate better results

In Figs. 6.4a and b, the distributions of two classes, which are shown with the red dot and blue circle, overlap with each other to a large extent. In contrast, Fig. 6.4c shows that the new representations obtained by JOLL4R are more separable. In particular, a majority of the samples in the cordectomy class lying in the upper-left can be easily separated. Hence, the new representations learned are more discriminative, which demonstrates the effectiveness of the proposed JOLL4R approach.

6.5.2   Classifier in JOLL4R

Even though nearest neighbor (1-NN) is used for the classification in JOLL4R, other classifiers, such as support vector machine (SVM), can be used. Table 6.6 shows the performance difference when linear SVM is used (same dataset as in Sect. 6.4.1). Additionally, since JOLL4R uses feature matrices as input, this model is also applicable to the fusion of other modalities other than audio.

6.5.3 Extension to Fusion of More Audios

Although joint learning is mainly used for the fusion of two audios in this chapter, JOLL4R can be easily extended to fuse more audios, in which the numbers of parameters to be optimized is twice of the audio number.

$$\min_{\mathbf{W_i},\mathbf{M}} \left\| \sum_{i=1}^{m} \left(\frac{1}{m}\mathbf{X_i}^{\mathrm{T}}\mathbf{W_i}\right) - \left(\mathbf{Y} + \mathbf{E} \odot \mathbf{M}\right) \right\|_F^2 + \sum_{i=1}^{m} \lambda_{i1} \|\mathbf{W_i}\|_F^2$$

$$+ \sum_{i=1}^{m} \lambda_{i2} \|\mathbf{W_i}\|_* \quad \text{s.t.} \quad \mathbf{M} \geqslant \mathbf{0} \tag{6.26}$$

Note that m is the audio number for fusion and W_i is the projection matrix for the ith audio. To alleviate the efforts in parameter optimization, parameter λ_{i1}, which controls the weight of each audio, can be adjusted adaptively. For instance, we may adopt the trick in Feng et al. (2012) to update the weights by solving the following problem:

$$\min_{\mathbf{W_i},\mathbf{M}} \left\| \sum_{i=1}^{m} \left(\frac{1}{m}\mathbf{X_i}^{\mathrm{T}}\mathbf{W_i}\right) - \left(\mathbf{Y} + \mathbf{E} \odot \mathbf{M}\right) \right\|_F^2 + \sum_{i=1}^{m} \lambda_{i1}^{\gamma} \|\mathbf{W_i}\|_F^2 + \sum_{i=1}^{m} \lambda_{i2} \|\mathbf{W_i}\|_*$$

$$\text{s.t.} \quad \mathbf{M} \geqslant \mathbf{0}, \ \sum_{i=1}^{m} \lambda_{i1} = 1, \lambda_{i1} > 0,$$

$$\tag{6.27}$$

where γ is added to avoid trivial solution. The parameter λ_{i1} is then updated by Eq. (6.28).

$$\lambda_{i1}^+ = \frac{\left(1/tr\left(\mathbf{W_i}^{\mathrm{T}}\mathbf{W_i}\right)\right)^{1/(\gamma-1)}}{\sum\limits_{j=1}^{m} \left(1/tr\left(\mathbf{W_j}^{\mathrm{T}}\mathbf{W_j}\right)\right)^{1/(\gamma-1)}} \tag{6.28}$$

In this way, the number of parameters to be optimized is reduced by half.

6.6 Summary

In this chapter, we propose a regression based model JOLL4R to fuse features from two different audios for voice based disease detection. Four key factors contribute to the success of JOLL4R. Firstly, the fusing model couples the regression losses from two views together to adjust the weights adaptively so that the more discriminative view can be emphasized in the final classification. Secondly, the ε-dragging technique facilitates to construct flexible regression targets and to enlarge the margins between different classes. Thirdly, the low-rank regularization is used to explore the underlying correlation structures between classes and the Tikhonov regularization term is added to avoid overfitting. Finally, the ADASYN technique is employed to handle the class imbalance problem so that samples with diseases can be detected with a higher accuracy. Experimental results on two disease detection tasks, each with six types of fusion, demonstrate the superior performance of JOLL4R, comparing with other kinds of fusion models and methods used on a single view.

Our algorithm may provide motivation to explore model based fusion for detecting pathological voice of other diseases. However, there is also limitation for this model, such as the demand for parameter optimization. In the future, we may investigate the fusion of more views for the detection and attempt to explore shared and view-specific structures for the regression based fusion. Besides, we may try to alleviate the efforts for parameter optimization further and also plan to collect more samples from patients to achieve better results.

References

Al-nasheri, A., Muhammad, G., Alsulaiman, M., Ali, Z., Mesallam, T. A., Farahat, M., Malki, K. H., & Bencherif, M. A. (2017). An investigation of multidimensional voice program parameters in three different databases for voice pathology detection and classification. *J. Voice, 31*, 113 –e 9.

Arias-Londono, J. D., Godino-Llorente, J. I., Saenz-Lechn, N., Osma-Ruiz, V., & Castellanos-Dominguez, G. (2010). An improved method for voice pathology detection by means of a HMM-based feature space transformation. *Pattern Recogn., 43*, 3100 – 3112.

Barry, W. J., & Putzer, M. Saarbrucken voice database, institute of phonetics. http://www.stimmdatenbank.coli.uni-saarland.de/.

Brabanter, K. D., Karsmakers, P., Brabanter, J. D., Suykens, J., & Moor, B. D. (2012). Confidence bands for least squares support vector machine classifiers: A regression approach. *Pattern Recogn., 45*, 2280 – 2287. Brain Decoding.

Cai, X., Ding, C., Nie, F., & Huang, H. (2013). On the equivalent of lowrank linear regressions and linear discriminant analysis based regressions. In *Proceedings of the 19th ACM SIGKDD international conference on Knowledge discovery and data mining* (pp. 1124–1132). ACM.

Cao, P., Liu, X., Yang, J., Zhao, D., Huang, M., & Zaiane, O. (2018). $l_{2,1}- l_1$ regularized nonlinear multi-task representation learning based cognitive performance prediction of Alzheimer's disease. *Pattern Recogn., 79*, 195 – 215.

Fang, X., Xu, Y., Li, X., Lai, Z., Wong, W. K., & Fang, B. (2018). Regularized label relaxation linear regression. *IEEE Transactions on Neural Networks, 29*, 1006–1018.

Feng, Q., & Zhou, Y. (2016). Kernel combined sparse representation for disease recognition. *IEEE Trans. Multimedia, 18*, 1956–1968.

Feng, Y., Xiao, J., Zhuang, Y., & Liu, X. (2012). Adaptive unsupervised multiview feature selection for visual concept recognition. In *Asian Conference on Computer Vision* (pp. 343–357). Springer.

Godino-Llorente, J. I., Gomez-Vilda, P., & Blanco-Velasco, M. (2006). Dimensionality reduction of a pathological voice quality assessment system based on Gaussian mixture models and short-term cepstral parameters. *IEEE Trans. Biomed. Eng., 53*, 1943–1953.

Grave, E., Obozinski, G. R., & Bach, F. R. (2011). Trace lasso: a trace norm regularization for correlated designs. In *Advances in Neural Information Processing Systems* (pp. 2187–2195).

He, H., Bai, Y., Garcia, E. A., & Li, S. (2008). ADASYN: Adaptive synthetic sampling approach for imbalanced learning. In *Neural Networks, 2008. IJCNN 2008. (IEEE World Congress on Computational Intelligence). IEEE International Joint Conference on* (pp. 1322–1328). IEEE.

Hoerl, A. E., & Kennard, R. W. (1970). Ridge regression: Biased estimation for nonorthogonal problems. *Technometrics, 12*, 55–67.

Lopez-de Ipina, K., Alonso, J.-B., Travieso, C. M., Sole-Casals, J., Egiraun, H., Faundez-Zanuy, M., Ezeiza, A., Barroso, N., Ecay-Torres, M., MartinezLage, P. et al. (2013). On the selection of non-invasive methods based on speech analysis oriented to automatic Alzheimer disease diagnosis. *Sensors, 13*, 6730–6745.

Lai, Z., Mo, D., Wen, J., Shen, L., & Wong, W. K. (2019). Generalized robust regression for jointly sparse subspace learning. *IEEE Transactions on Circuits and Systems for Video Technology, 29*, 756–772.

Lai, Z., Mo, D., Wong, W. K., Xu, Y., Miao, D., & Zhang, D. (2018). Robust discriminant regression for feature extraction. *IEEE Transactions on Systems, Man, and Cybernetics, 48*, 2472–2484.

Lai, Z., Wong, W. K., Xu, Y., Yang, J., & Zhang, D. (2016). Approximate orthogonal sparse embedding for dimensionality reduction. *IEEE Transactions on Neural Networks, 27*, 723–735.

Levina, E., & Bickel, P. J. (2005). Maximum likelihood estimation of intrinsic dimension. In *Advances in neural information processing systems* (pp. 777 – 784).

Little, M. A., McSharry, P. E., Hunter, E. J., Spielman, J., Ramig, L. O. et al. (2009). Suitability of dysphonia measurements for telemonitoring of Parkinson's disease. *IEEE Trans. Biomed. Eng., 56*, 1015–1022.

Little, M. A., McSharry, P. E., Roberts, S. J., Costello, D. A., & Moroz, I. M. (2007). Exploiting nonlinear recurrence and fractal scaling properties for voice disorder detection. *Biomed. Eng. Online, 6*, 23.

Ludlow, C., Bassich, C., Connor, N., Coulter, D., Lee, Y., Baer, T., Sasaki, C., & Harris, K. (1987). The validity of using phonatory jitter and shimmer to detect laryngeal pathology. In *Laryngeal function in phonation and respiration* (pp. 492–508). College-Hill Press, Boston.

Maciel, C. D., Guido, R. C., Fonseca, E. S., Montagnoli, A. N., & Vieira, L. S. (2007). Autoregressive decomposition and pole tracking applied to vocal fold nodule signals. *Pattern Recogn. Lett., 28*, 1360–1367.

Martinez, D., Lleida, E., Ortega, A., & Miguel, A. (2012a). Score level versus audio level fusion for voice pathology detection on the Saarbrucken Voice Database. In *Advances in Speech and Language Technologies for Iberian Languages* (pp. 110–120). Berlin, Heidelberg: Springer Berlin Heidelberg.

Martinez, D., Lleida, E., Ortega, A., Miguel, A., & Villalba, J. (2012b). Voice pathology detection on the Saarbrucken Voice Database with calibration and fusion of scores using multifocal toolkit. In *Advances in Speech and Language Technologies for Iberian Languages* (pp. 99–109). Berlin, Heidelberg: Springer Berlin Heidelberg.

Maryn, Y., Corthals, P., Van Cauwenberge, P., Roy, N., & De Bodt, M. (2010). Toward improved ecological validity in the acoustic measurement of overall voice quality: combining continuous speech and sustained vowels. *J. Voice, 24*, 540–555.

Mazumder, R., Hastie, T., & Tibshirani, R. (2010). Spectral regularization algorithms for learning large incomplete matrices. *J. Mach. Learn. Res.*, *11*, 2287–2322.

Mekyska, J., Smekal, Z., Galaz, Z., Mzourek, Z., Rektorova, I., Faundez-Zanuy, M., & Lopez-de Ipina, K. (2016). Perceptual features as markers of Parkinson's disease: the issue of clinical interpretability. In *Recent Advances in Nonlinear Speech Processing* (pp. 83–91). Springer.

Muhammad, G., Alsulaiman, M., Ali, Z., Mesallam, T. A., Farahat, M., Malki, K. H., Al-nasheri, A., & Bencherif, M. A. (2017). Voice pathology detection using interlaced derivative pattern on glottal source excitation. *Biomed. Signal Process. Control*, *31*, 156–164.

Oguz, H., Demirci, M., Safak, M. A., Arslan, N., Islam, A., & Kargin, S. (2007). Effects of unilateral vocal cord paralysis on objective voice measures obtained by Praat. *Eur. Arch. Oto-Rhino-Laryn.*, *264*, 257–261.

Orozco-Arroyave, J., Honig, F., Arias-Londono, J., Vargas-Bonilla, J., Daqrouq, K., Skodda, S., Rusz, J., & Noth, E. (2016). Automatic detection of Parkinson's disease in running speech spoken in three different languages. *J. Acoust. Soc. Am.*, *139*, 481–500.

Peng, C., Kang, Z., Xu, F., Chen, Y., & Cheng, Q. (2017). Image projection ridge regression for subspace clustering. *IEEE Signal Process. Lett.*, *24*, 991 –995.

Saudi, A. S. M., Youssif, A. A., & Ghalwash, A. Z. (2012). Computer aided recognition of vocal folds disorders by means of RASTA-PLP. *Comput. Inf. Sci.*, *5*, 39.

Shin, D., Lee, H. S., & Kim, D. (2007). Illumination-robust face recognition using ridge regressive bilinear models. *Pattern Recogn. Lett.*, *29*, 49–58.

Trinh, D. H., Luong, M., Rocchisani, J.-M., Pham, C. D., & Dibos, F. (2011). Medical image denoising using kernel ridge regression. In *Image Processing (ICIP), 2011 18th IEEE International Conference on* (pp. 1597–1600). IEEE.

Tsanas, A. (2012). *Accurate telemonitoring of Parkinson's disease symptom severity using nonlinear speech signal processing and statistical machine learning*. Ph.D. thesis University of Oxford.

Tsanas, A., Little, M. A., McSharry, P. E., & Ramig, L. O. (2010). Accurate telemonitoring of Parkinson's disease progression by noninvasive speech tests. *IEEE Trans. Biomed. Eng.*, *57*, 884–893.

Tsanas, A., Little, M. A., McSharry, P. E., Spielman, J., & Ramig, L. O. (2012). Novel speech signal processing algorithms for high-accuracy classification of Parkinson's disease. *IEEE Trans. Biomed. Eng.*, *59*, 1264–1271.

Vaiciukynas, E., Verikas, A., Gelzinis, A., Bacauskiene, M., Kons, Z., Satt, A., & Hoory, R. (2014). Fusion of voice signal information for detection of mild laryngeal pathology. *Appl. Soft. Comput.*, *18*, 91–103.

Vaiciukynas, E., Verikas, A., Gelzinis, A., Bacauskiene, M., Vaskevicius, K., Uloza, V., Padervinskis, E., & Ciceliene, J. (2016). Fusing various audio feature sets for detection of Parkinson's disease from sustained voice and speech recordings. In *International Conference on Speech and Computer* (pp. 328 – 337). Springer.

Van Gestel, T., Suykens, J. A., Lanckriet, G., Lambrechts, A., De Moor, B., & Vandewalle, J. (2002). Bayesian framework for least-squares support vector machine classifiers, Gaussian processes, and kernel Fisher discriminant analysis. *Neural Comput.*, *14*, 1115–1147.

Wong, W. K., Lai, Z., Wen, J., Fang, X., & Lu, Y. (2017). Low-rank embedding for robust image feature extraction. *IEEE Transactions on Image Processing*, *26*, 2905–2917.

Wright, J., Yang, A. Y., Ganesh, A., Sastry, S. S., & Ma, Y. (2009). Robust face recognition via sparse representation. *IEEE Trans. Pattern Anal. Mach. Intell.*, *31*, 210–227.

Wu, K., Zhang, D., Lu, G., & Guo, Z. (2019). Joint learning for voice based disease detection. *Pattern Recogn.*, *87*, 130–139.

Xiang, S., Nie, F., Meng, G., Pan, C., & Zhang, C. (2012). Discriminative least squares regression for multiclass classification and feature selection. *IEEE Trans. Neural Netw. Learn.*, *23*, 1738–1754.

Xue, H., Chen, S., & Yang, Q. (2009). Discriminatively regularized least-squares classification. *Pattern Recogn.*, *42*, 93–104.

Yumoto, E., Gould, W. J., & Baer, T. (1982). Harmonics-to-noise ratio as an index of the degree of hoarseness. *J. Acoust. Soc. Am.*, *71*, 1544–1550.

Zhang, X.-Y., Wang, L., Xiang, S., & Liu, C.-L. (2015). Retargeted least squares regression algorithm. *IEEE Trans. Neural Netw. Learn.*, *26*, 2206–2213.

Zhang, Z., Lai, Z., Xu, Y., Shao, L., Wu, J., & Xie, G.-S. (2017). Discriminative elastic-net regularized linear regression. *IEEE Trans. Image Process.*, *26*, 1466–1481.

Zou, H., & Hastie, T. (2005). Regularization and variable selection via the elastic net. *J. R. Stat. Soc. Ser. B-Stat. Methodol.*, *67*, 301–320.

Chapter 7
Robust Multi-View Discriminative Learning for Voice Based Disease Detection

Abstract Voice analysis is a non-invasive, painless, and convenient alternative for disease detection. Despite many existing methods for voice based pathology detection, they generally consider a single audio, even though different audios provide complementary information and a fusion of them would contribute to improving the classification performance. In this chapter, a robust multi-view model ROME-DLR (RObust Multi-viEw Discriminative learning based on Label Relaxed regression) is proposed. First, a shared-specific structure is assumed to model the correlation between different views. Then we enlarge the margins between different classes by relaxing the conventional rigid zero-one regression targets to learn more discriminative projections. Considering possible outliers in real-world data, $l_{2,1}$ norm is introduced to the regression loss term to seek more robust representations. Experimental results on two disease detection tasks demonstrate the effectiveness and superiority of our fusion approach compared with the state-of-the-art methods.

Keywords Discriminative learning · Multi-view · Robust · Voice based pathology detection

7.1 Introduction

Compared with advanced diagnostic tools like laryngoscope and endoscope, voice analysis is an alternative that is non-invasive, painless, and convenient. Therefore, researchers are motivated to employ voice analysis to detect diseases like Parkinson's disease (PD) (Tsanas et al. 2012), Alzheimer's disease (Lopez-de Ipina et al. 2013), vocal cord paralysis (Saudi et al. 2012), and vocal cord nodule (Oguz et al. 2007). In (Tsanas et al. 2010), Tsanas et al. even used voice analysis to assess the severity of PD.

In voice based disease detection, a variety of discriminative features are designed to classify healthy and pathological voice (Maciel et al. 2007; Arias-Londono et al. 2010). These features can generally be categorized into three classes. Features in the first category are to quantify the periodicity extent of voice signal. For pathological voice, the vibration of vocal folds tends to deviate from periodicity. Jitter and

© Springer Nature Singapore Pte Ltd. 2020
D. Zhang, K. Wu, *Pathological Voice Analysis*,
https://doi.org/10.1007/978-981-32-9196-6_7

shimmer, which describe the perturbations of the fundamental frequency and amplitude over periods, respectively, are the two most representative features in this class (Ludlow et al. 1987). Other features describing the periodicity extent include glottal quotient (Tsanas 2012), recurrence period density entropy (Little et al. 2007), and pitch period entropy (Little et al. 2009). Secondly, there are features assessing the noise extent in voice caused by incomplete glottal closures, among which harmonics to noise ratio (Yumoto et al. 1982) and noise to harmonics ratio (Jotz et al. 2002) are classic features in this class. In the third category, features devised for speech and speaker recognition are adopted, such as Mel-frequency cepstral coefficients (MFCC) (Garcia and Garcia 2003), linear prediction coefficients (LPC) (Childers and Bae 1992), and linear prediction cepstral coefficients (LPCC) (Saldanha et al. 2014). Particularly, study in (Godino-Llorente et al. 2006; Godino-Llorente and Gomez-Vilda 2004) demonstrated MFCC has a good degree of reliability for disease detection. In voice analysis, the most frequently adopted vocal tests are running speech (Orozco-Arroyave et al. 2016) and sustained vowels (Shi et al. 2014). Since running speech is often coupled with confounding effects, most studies use a single vowel of normal pitch for analysis, in which patients are asked to pronounce a vowel and sustain it as long as possible (Shi et al. 2014).

Despite the many approaches developed for voice based disease detection, most of them use a single audio, in which the dominant one is the sustained vowel /a/ produced with a normal pitch. Nevertheless, it is known that different views (modalities) of the same instance provide complementary information and an exploitation of multi-view (multi-modality) data is often beneficial for classification tasks (Li et al. 2017; Hu et al. 2015; Shi et al. 2014). In voice analysis, it is natural to hypothesize that when a certain sample cannot be classified with features from one audio, it may be correctly detected by another audio. Moreover, it is difficult to detect a patient accurately with a single audio, whereas a combination of multi-audio may result in an accurate diagnosis. Therefore, an effective exploitation of the complementary information from multi-audio may be advantageous for disease detection.

Previous literature for voice based disease detection consists of three levels of fusion: (1) audio-level fusion, which concatenates multi-audios into a single recording (Maryn et al. 2010; Martinez et al. 2012a); (2) feature-level fusion that concatenates feature vectors extracted from different audios into a single vector for classification (Vaiciukynas et al. 2014); (3) the mostly used decision-level fusion that combines the scores (or classification results) obtained from different audios (Martinez et al. 2012a, b; Vaiciukynas et al. 2014, 2016). Even though audio-level and feature-level fusions are quite simple, it may not be effective since (1) the differences among different audios are ignored and (2) the cross correlations among different audios are not considered. Decision-level fusion, which was shown to outperform the first two types of fusion (Martinez et al. 2012a; Vaiciukynas et al. 2014), is time-consuming due to the training of multiple classifiers. Hence, it is necessary to investigate a new type of fusion for voice based disease detection.

Here we propose a robust multi-view discriminative learning model. Since each audio, in fact, presents a "view" for disease detection, the proposed learning model using multi-audio is referred as a multi-view model. Starting from extending the conventional least square regression model to the multi-view version, we then relax the traditional binary regression targets to increase flexibility and to enlarge the margins between different classes so that more discriminative transformation matrices can be learned. Next, the shared-specific structure in multi-view data is uncovered by redesigning the transformation matrices as the weighted sum of the shared and view-specific components. Finally, instead of using the Frobenius norm, we employ the $l_{2,1}$-norm based prediction loss term to reduce the influence of outliers. It is worthwhile to note that the number of views for fusion is not restricted in our method. Experiments demonstrate the great performance of the proposed multi-view model.

The rest of this chapter is organized as follows. Section 7.2 presents our proposed robust multi-view discriminative learning algorithm. In Sects. 7.3 and 7.4, experimental results and discussions are given, respectively. Finally, we conclude this chapter and present the future work in Sect. 7.5.

7.2 Proposed Method

7.2.1 Notation

In this chapter, matrices and column vectors are denoted by bold uppercase and bold lowercase letters, respectively. A^{T} represents the transposed matrix of A and I is an identity matrix. $\|\mathbf{A}\|_F^2 = tr(\mathbf{A}^{\mathrm{T}}\mathbf{A}) = tr(\mathbf{A}\mathbf{A}^{\mathrm{T}})$ stands for the square of the Frobenius norm of matrix A, in which $tr(\cdot)$ is the trace operator. For an arbitrary matrix $A \in \mathrm{R}^{p \times q}$, its $l_{2,1}$-norm is defined as $\|\mathbf{A}\|_{2,1} = \sum_{i=1}^{p} \sqrt{\sum_{j=1}^{q} a_{ij}^2}$, where a_{ij} is the (i,j)th entry of A.

7.2.2 The Objective Function

Given a centered multi-view dataset consisting of n training instances from m views, we denote the feature matrix of each view i ($i = 1, 2, \ldots, m$) as $X_i \in \mathrm{R}^{d \times n}$, where d is the feature dimensionality. The labels for all the training samples are represented by $Y \in \mathrm{R}^{n \times c}$, with c being the number of classes. Each row of Y is a binary vector $[0, \cdots, 0, 1, 0, \cdots, 0]$. When a sample is from the kth class ($k = 1, 2, \cdots, c$), then only the kth entry of the binary vector is assigned to one.

To begin with, a multi-view model based on the widely used Least Square Regression (LSR) is formulated.

$$\min_{\mathbf{W_i}} \sum_{i=1}^{m} \left(\left\| \mathbf{Y} - \mathbf{X_i}^{\mathrm{T}}\mathbf{W_i} \right\|_F^2 + \beta \|\mathbf{W_i}\|_F^2 \right). \tag{7.1}$$

Here, $W_i \in \mathbf{R}^{d \times c}$ ($i = 1, 2, \cdots, m$) is a projection matrix and the Tikhonov regularization term is added to reduce the variance of the model by shrinking the coefficients in W_i. Even though Eq. (7.1) is simple and yet effective for some applications (Shin et al. 2007), it has three main disadvantages. First of all, the correlation between different views is neglected. It can be easily proved that Eq. (7.1) yields the same results as do view-by-view regressions (Izenman 2008). As a result, nothing is gained by estimating the projections jointly, even though the feature matrices of different views may be correlated. Secondly, the zero-one entries in the label matrix Y limit the power of LSR for data classification since the zero-one targets are too rigid to learn (Zhang et al. 2015). Thirdly, noise and outliers in real-world data may result in overfitting when using Frobenius norm in the regression term. In order to learn discriminative and robust representations for multi-view data, we argue that the above three weaknesses should be handled.

Shared-Specific Structures We first elaborate on how to utilize the correlation among different views. On one hand, it is reasonable to assume that feature vectors extracted from different views of the same sample may share some similarity. Therefore, the multiple projection matrices should be somewhat similar, using such prior can help to increase the stability of our model. On the other hand, those different views may hold their specific and complementary distinctiveness so that their projection matrices should have diversity and flexibility. Therefore, exploring the shared-specific structures is beneficial to learn stable and accurate projections for subsequent classification. The idea of shared-specific structures has been explored from different perspectives in the literature (Yang et al. 2012; Li et al. 2017; Hu et al. 2015). For instance, some researchers designed to explore the shared-specific coding vectors in linear representation learning (Yang et al. 2012; Li et al. 2017). In Hu et al. (2015), the shared-specific structures were used in the projected subspace under the framework of LSR. We propose the following model to regularize the projection matrices so that the shared-specific structures in the multi-view data are uncovered.

$$\min_{\mathbf{W_i}, \mathbf{W_0}} \sum_{i=1}^{m} \left(\left\| \mathbf{Y} - \mathbf{X_i}^{\mathrm{T}}(\lambda\mathbf{W_0} + (1-\lambda)\mathbf{W_i}) \right\|_F^2 + \beta \|\mathbf{W_i}\|_F^2 \right) + \alpha \|\mathbf{W_0}\|_F^2$$

$$+ \tau \left\| \mathbf{W_0} - \frac{1}{m}\sum_{i=1}^{m}\mathbf{W_i} \right\|_F^2, \tag{7.2}$$

where $W_0 \in \mathbf{R}^{d \times c}$ and W_i denote the projection matrices for shared and view-specific components, respectively. The last term in Eq. (7.2) is added to enforce the average W_i ($i = 1, 2, \cdots, m$) of all views to be similar to the shared projection. $\lambda \in [0,1]$ and $\tau \geq 0$ are two constants that balance the learned shared and specific cues. A larger λ indicates a higher weight on the shared structure and lower weight on the view-specific ones. Similarly, a large τ encourages more emphasis on the shared component. With the first and last terms in Eq. (7.2), we are able to uncover the shared-specific structures more flexibly.

Label Relaxation Secondly, the zero-one entries in the label matrix Y are too rigid so that the learned projection matrices are less discriminative, especially for multi-class classification tasks. To make LSR based classification model more effective, some studies revised the loss function of LSR, such as the model of least squares support vector machine in Gestel et al. (2002) and Brabanter et al. (2012) and the discriminatively regularized LSR in Xue et al. (2009). Other researchers attempted to modify the binary regression targets in LSR so that the targets were less rigid. For instance, it was proposed in Zhang et al. (2015) to learn the regression targets rather than using the binary label directly. In Xiang et al. (2012), Xiang et al. put forward a ε-dragging technique to revise the regression targets for discriminative LSR.

Assume the binary label matrix $\mathbf{Y} = [\mathbf{y_1}^T, \mathbf{y_2}^T, \cdots, \mathbf{y_n}^T]^T$, where $y_i \in \mathbb{R}^{1 \times c}$ is a row vector indicating the class label of the ith instance. For each y_i from the kth class, the ε ε-dragging technique is to drag the binary entries far away along two opposite directions so that the kth entry in y_i with "1" becomes "$1 + \epsilon_{i1}$" and other entries with "0"s are changed to "$-\epsilon_{i0}^j$," where "ϵ_{i1}" and "ϵ_{i0}^j" are positive slack variables ($i \in \{1, \cdots, n\}, j \in \{1, \cdots, c, j \neq k\}$). In this way, the label distance between two data points from different classes is enlarged and discriminative projection matrices, which is generally desired for classification tasks, can be obtained. With the ε-dragging technique, we relax the label matrix Y in Eq. (7.2) as follows:

$$\min_{\mathbf{W_i}, \mathbf{W_0}, \mathbf{M_i}} \sum_{i=1}^{m} \left(\left\| \left(\mathbf{Y} + \mathbf{E} \odot \mathbf{M_i} \right) - \mathbf{X_i}^T (\lambda \mathbf{W_0} + (1 - \lambda) \mathbf{W_i}) \right\|_F^2 + \beta \|\mathbf{W_i}\|_F^2 \right)$$

$$+ \alpha \|\mathbf{W_0}\|_F^2 + \tau \left\| \mathbf{W_0} - \frac{1}{m} \sum_{i=1}^{m} \mathbf{W_i} \right\|_F^2 \quad \text{s.t.} \quad \mathbf{M_i} \geq \mathbf{0}$$

$$(7.3)$$

where the relaxed label matrix is constructed by $\mathbf{Y} + \mathbf{E} \odot \mathbf{M_i}$. Here $\mathbf{M_i}$ is a nonnegative matrix to be learned and E is a constant matrix defined as

$$E_{pq} = \begin{cases} +1 & \text{if } Y_{pq} = 1 \\ -1 & \text{if } Y_{pq} = 0 \end{cases} \quad (7.4)$$

Adding the term $\mathbf{Y} + \mathbf{E} \odot \mathbf{M_i}$ relaxes the strict binary regression target matrix to some soft extents to gain more flexibility to fit the data. In addition, the design of the signs in E and the nonnegativity constraint on $\mathbf{M_i}$ guarantees that the distance between any two data points of different classes in $\mathbf{Y} + \mathbf{E} \odot \mathbf{M_i}$ is larger than the corresponding distance in $\mathbf{Y}$. The enlarged distance then makes the learned projections more discriminative. Note that we do not set relaxed label to be equal for all views, but instead we learn a relaxation-related matrix $\mathbf{M_i}$ for each view. Clearly, the kind of design makes our approach more flexible.

$l_{2,1}$-**norm Based Robust Regression** The third weakness in Eq. (7.1) is that it cannot handle outliers well. With the squared residue error in the form of Frobenius norm, a few outliers with large errors can easily dominate the objective function. For this reason, a robust loss function is desired. According to the definition of $l_{2,1}$-norm in Sect. 7.2.1, the residue error is not squared if we replace the Frobenius norm with the $l_{2,1}$-norm (Kong et al. 2011; Ren et al. 2012). In this way, our model can be more robust since the large errors caused by outliers do not dominate the loss function. The final objective function of our multi-view learning model is presented as below.

$$\min_{\mathbf{W_i}, \mathbf{W_0}, \mathbf{M_i}} \sum_{i=1}^{m} \left(\left\| \left(\mathbf{Y} + \mathbf{E} \odot \mathbf{M_i} \right) - \mathbf{X_i}^{\mathrm{T}} (\lambda \mathbf{W_0} + (1 - \lambda) \mathbf{W_i} \right\|_{2,1} + \beta \|\mathbf{W_i}\|_F^2 \right)$$
$$+ \alpha \|\mathbf{W_0}\|_F^2 + \tau \left\| \mathbf{W_0} - \frac{1}{m} \sum_{i=1}^{m} \mathbf{W_i} \right\|_F^2 \quad \text{s.t.} \quad \mathbf{M_i} \geqslant \mathbf{0}. \quad (7.5)$$

Thereafter, we refer the proposed model as RObust Multi-viEw Discriminative learning based on Label Relaxed regression (ROME-DLR).

7.2.3   Optimization of ROME-DLR

In this section, we tackle the $l_{2,1}$-norm minimization problem in Eq. (7.5) by proposing an efficient algorithm via the Augmented Lagrangian method (ALM) (Ghasemishabankareh et al. 2016). According to ALM, slack variables $B_i \in \mathbb{R}^{n \times c} (i = 1, 2, \ldots, m)$ are introduced to replace $(\mathbf{Y} + \mathbf{E} \odot \mathbf{M_i}) - \mathbf{X_i}^{\mathrm{T}} (\lambda \mathbf{W_0} + (1 - \lambda) \mathbf{W_i})$ so that the objective function in Eq. (7.5) can be rewritten as

$$\min_{\mathbf{W_i}, \mathbf{W_0}, \mathbf{M_i}, \mathbf{B_i}} \sum_{i=1}^{m} \left(\|\mathbf{B_i}\|_{2,1} + \beta \|\mathbf{W_i}\|_F^2 \right) + \alpha \|\mathbf{W_0}\|_F^2 + \tau \left\| \mathbf{W_0} - \frac{1}{m} \sum_{i=1}^{m} \mathbf{W_i} \right\|_F^2. \quad (7.6)$$
$$\text{s.t.} \quad \mathbf{M_i} \geqslant \mathbf{0}; \quad \mathbf{B_i} = \mathbf{Y} + \mathbf{E} \odot \mathbf{M_i} - \mathbf{X_i}^{\mathrm{T}} (\lambda \mathbf{W_0} + (1 - \lambda) \mathbf{W_i}),$$

The objective function in Eq. (7.6) can be further transformed into the following problem:

$$\min_{\mathbf{W_i}, \mathbf{W_0}, \mathbf{M_i}, \mathbf{B_i}, \mathbf{C_i}} \sum_{i=1}^{m} \left(\frac{\mu}{2} \left\| \mathbf{B_i} - \left(\mathbf{Y} + \mathbf{E} \odot \mathbf{M_i} \right) + \mathbf{X_i}^{\mathrm{T}} (\lambda \mathbf{W_0} + (1 - \lambda) \mathbf{W_i}) + \frac{\mathbf{C_i}}{\mu} \right\|_F^2 \right.$$
$$+ \|\mathbf{B_i}\|_{2,1} + \beta \|\mathbf{W_i}\|_F^2 \right) + \alpha \|\mathbf{W_0}\|_F^2$$
$$+ \tau \left\| \mathbf{W_0} - \frac{1}{m} \sum_{i=1}^{m} \mathbf{W_i} \right\|_F^2 \quad \text{s.t.} \quad \mathbf{M_i} \geqslant \mathbf{0}, , \quad (7.7)$$

where $C_i \in \mathbb{R}^{n \times c}$ is Lagrange multiplier and $\mu > 0$ is the penalty parameter. We solve the problem Eq. (7.7) by iteratively updating W_i, W_0, M_i, B_i, and C_i with the following steps.

STEP 1 *Update W_i.* Fix other variables, the optimization solution of Eq. (7.7) over W_i equals to the following problem, where terms irrelevant to W_i are discarded.

$$\min_{\mathbf{W_i}} \frac{\mu}{2} \left\| \mathbf{B_i} - \left(\mathbf{Y} + \mathbf{E} \odot \mathbf{M_i} \right) + \mathbf{X_i}^{\mathrm{T}}(\lambda \mathbf{W_0} + (1 - \lambda)\mathbf{W_i}) + \frac{\mathbf{C_i}}{\mu} \right\|_F^2$$
$$+ \beta \|\mathbf{W_i}\|_F^2 + \tau \left\| \mathbf{W_0} - \frac{1}{m} \sum_{i=1}^m \mathbf{W_i} \right\|_F^2. \tag{7.8}$$

By setting the derivation of Eq. (7.8) with respect to W_i to zero, the optimal W_i can be obtained as follows:

$$\mathbf{W_i^+} = \left(\mu(1 - \lambda)^2 \mathbf{X_i} \mathbf{X_i}^{\mathrm{T}} + \left(2\beta + \frac{2\tau}{m} \right) \mathbf{I} \right)^{-1} \left(-\mu(1 - \lambda)\mathbf{X_i} \left(\mathbf{B_i} - \left(\mathbf{Y} + \mathbf{E} \odot \mathbf{M_i} \right) \right. \right.$$
$$\left. \left. + \lambda \mathbf{X_i}^{\mathrm{T}} \mathbf{W_0} + \frac{\mathbf{C_i}}{\mu} \right) + \frac{2\tau}{m} \left(\mathbf{W_0} - \frac{1}{m} \sum_{k=1, k \neq i}^m \mathbf{W_k} \right) \right). \tag{7.9}$$

STEP 2 *Update W_0.* Keeping other variables fixed, the problem to be solved is

$$\min_{\mathbf{W_0}} \sum_{i=1}^m \left\| \frac{\mu}{2} \mathbf{B_i} - \left(\mathbf{Y} + \mathbf{E} \odot \mathbf{M_i} \right) + \mathbf{X_i}^{\mathrm{T}}(\lambda \mathbf{W_0} + (1 - \lambda)\mathbf{W_i}) \right.$$
$$\left. + \frac{\mathbf{C_i}}{\mu} \right\|_F^2 + \alpha \|\mathbf{W_0}\|_F^2 + \tau \left\| \mathbf{W_0} - \frac{1}{m} \sum_{i=1}^m \mathbf{W_i} \right\|_F^2. \tag{7.10}$$

Similarly, after setting the derivative of the objective function in Eq. (7.10) with respect to W_0 to zero, we can update W_0 by

$$\mathbf{W_0^+} = \left(\sum_{i=1}^m (\mu\lambda^2 \mathbf{X_i} \mathbf{X_i}^{\mathrm{T}}) + (2\alpha + 2\tau)\mathbf{I} \right)^{-1} \left(-\sum_{i=1}^m \mu\lambda \mathbf{X_i} \left(\mathbf{B_i} - \left(\mathbf{Y} + \mathbf{E} \odot \mathbf{M_i} \right) \right. \right.$$
$$\left. \left. + (1 - \lambda)\mathbf{X_i}^{\mathrm{T}} \mathbf{W_i} + \frac{\mathbf{C_i}}{\mu} \right) + \frac{2\tau}{m} \sum_{i=1}^m \mathbf{W_i} \right). \tag{7.11}$$

STEP 3 *Update M_i.* When other variables are fixed, we have the following optimization problem:

$$\min_{\mathbf{M_i}} \frac{\mu}{2} \left\| \mathbf{B_i} - \left(\mathbf{Y} + \mathbf{E} \odot \mathbf{M_i} \right) + \mathbf{X_i}^{\mathrm{T}} (\lambda \mathbf{W_0} + (1 - \lambda) \mathbf{W_i}) + \frac{\mathbf{C_i}}{\mu} \right\|_F^2 \quad \text{s.t.} \quad \mathbf{M_i} \geqslant \mathbf{0}.$$

(7.12)

Let $\mathbf{Q_i} = \mathbf{B_i} - \mathbf{Y} + \mathbf{X_i}^{\mathrm{T}} (\lambda \mathbf{W_0} + (1 - \lambda) \mathbf{W_i}) + \frac{\mathbf{C_i}}{\mu}$, then Eq. (7.12) can be rewritten as

$$\min_{\mathbf{M_i}} \frac{\mu}{2} \left\| \mathbf{Q_i} - \mathbf{E} \odot \mathbf{M_i} \right\|_F^2 \quad \text{s.t.} \quad \mathbf{M_i} \geqslant \mathbf{0}.$$

(7.13)

According to the work in Xiang et al. (2012), the solution to Eq. (7.13) is

$$\mathbf{M_i^+} = \max \left(\mathbf{Q_i} \odot \mathbf{E}, \mathbf{0} \right).$$

(7.14)

STEP 4 *Update B_i.* Given fixed variables W_i, W_0, M_i, and C_i, the optimization problem of Eq. (7.7) can be reformulated to Eq. (7.15) at the step of updating B_i.

$$\min_{\mathbf{B_i}} \frac{\mu}{2} \left\| \mathbf{B_i} - \left(\mathbf{Y} + \mathbf{E} \odot \mathbf{M_i} \right) + \mathbf{X_i}^{\mathrm{T}} (\lambda \mathbf{W_0} + (1 - \lambda) \mathbf{W_i}) + \frac{\mathbf{C_i}}{\mu} \right\|_F^2$$
$$+ \left\| \mathbf{B_i} \right\|_{2,1}.$$

(7.15)

Denote $\mathbf{P_i} = \mathbf{Y} + \mathbf{E} \odot \mathbf{M_i} - \mathbf{X_i}^{\mathrm{T}} (\lambda \mathbf{W_0} + (1 - \lambda) \mathbf{W_i}) - \frac{\mathbf{C_i}}{\mu}$, then Eq. (7.15) can be simplified as below.

$$L(\mathbf{B_i}) = \min_{\mathbf{B_i}} \frac{\mu}{2} \left\| \mathbf{B_i} - \mathbf{P_i} \right\|_F^2 + \left\| \mathbf{B_i} \right\|_{2,1}$$

(7.16)

According to (Nie et al. 2010), we get the derivative of $L(B_i)$ with respect to B_i:

$$\frac{\partial L(\mathbf{B_i})}{\partial \mathbf{B_i}} = \mu (\mathbf{B_i} - \mathbf{P_i}) + 2 \mathbf{D_i} \mathbf{B_i},$$

(7.17)

where D_i is a diagonal matrix with the j-th diagonal element as $d_{jj} = \frac{1}{2 \|\mathbf{B_i}(j,:)\|_2}$. $B_i(j,:)$ represents the j-th row vector in B_i. Setting Eq. (7.17) to zero, we get the update of B_i in Eq. (7.18).

$$\mathbf{B_i^+} = (2 \mathbf{D_i} + \mu \mathbf{I})^{-1} (\mu \mathbf{P_i})$$

(7.18)

We continue to alternately solve for W_i, W_0, M_i, and B_i by Eqs. (7.9), (7.11), (7.14), and (7.18) until a maximum number of iterations is reached or a predefined threshold is reached.

STEP 5 *Update C_i.* The Lagrange multiplier C_i is updated by Eq. (7.19).

$$\mathbf{C}_i^+ = \mathbf{C}_i + \mu\left(\mathbf{B}_i - \left(\mathbf{Y} + \mathbf{E} \odot \mathbf{M}_i\right) + \mathbf{X}_i^T(\lambda\mathbf{W}_0 + (1 - \lambda)\mathbf{W}_i)\right). \tag{7.19}$$

For clarity, the algorithm to optimize ROME-DLR is described in Algorithm 7.1.

7.2.4   The Classification Rule of ROME-DLR

As presented in Sect. 7.3.1, the database we use for voice based disease detection has the problem of class imbalance, in which the number of healthy subjects is much larger than that of the samples with diseases. Hence, an oversampling method ADAptive SYNthetic sampling (ADASYN) (He et al. 2008) is conducted on the training feature matrices, which enables to generate synthetic samples for the minority class to compensate for the skewed distribution. Note that the synthetic samples are used for training only. The effect of ADASYN is discussed experimentally in Sect. 7.3.4.

Algorithm 7.1 Optimization of ROME-DLR
Input: Feature matrices: $X_i, i = 1, 2, \cdots, m$; Label matrix: Y; Constant Matrix: E;
  Initialization: Initialize W_i and $W_0 \in R^{d \times c}$ randomly; $M_i = \mathbf{0}_{n \times c}$; $B_i = \mathbf{0}_{n \times c}$;
$C_i = \mathbf{0}_{n \times c}$; $\mu = 0.1$, $\alpha > 0$, $\beta > 0$, $\tau > 0$, and $\lambda \in [0, 1]$.
  1: **while** not converged **do**
  2:   **while** not converged **do**
  3:     **Step 1** Update W_i ($i = 1, 2, \cdots, m$) by Eq. (7.9).
  4:     **Step 2** Update W_0 according to Eq. (7.11).
  5:     **Step 3** Update M_i ($i = 1, 2, \cdots, m$) by Eq. (7.14).
  6:     **Step 4** Update B_i ($i = 1, 2, \cdots, m$) by Eq. (7.18).
  7:   **end while**
  8:   **Step 5** Update C_i ($i = 1, 2, \cdots, m$) by Eq. (7.19).
  9: **end while**
  Output: The Optimal Projection Matrices: W_i and W_0.

In this section, the training feature set and test feature set of the ith view are denoted as X_i^{tr} and X_i^{te}, respectively. Y^{tr} is the label matrix for training samples. Assume the synthetic samples generated by using ADASYN on X_i^{tr} are represented by X_i^{sy}, then the final feature set of ith view used for training the ROME-DLR model is $X_{di}^{tr} = [X_i^{tr}, X_i^{sy}]$. Accordingly, the new label matrix is denoted as Y_d^{tr}.

Next, we input X_{di}^{tr} and Y_d^{tr} in Algorithm 7.1 to learn the projection matrices W_i and W_0, which are then used to transform the feature matrices of training samples X_{di}^{tr} and test samples X_i^{te} by Eqs. 7.20 and 7.21, respectively.

$$\mathbf{R}_i^{tr} = \left(\mathbf{X}_i^{tr}\right)^T(\lambda\mathbf{W_0} + (1 - \lambda)\mathbf{W_i}). \tag{7.20}$$

$$\mathbf{R}_i^{te} = \left(\mathbf{X}_i^{te}\right)^T(\lambda\mathbf{W_0} + (1 - \lambda)\mathbf{W_i}). \tag{7.21}$$

The final representation is formed by concatenating the transformed feature matrices R_i^{tr} (R_i^{te}) of all views together. Clearly, the dimensionality for each instance will be equal to $c \times m$. Eventually, the simple nearest neighbor (1-NN) classifier follows to make the final decision.

7.3   Experimental Results

7.3.1   Dataset and Experimental Setup

The database used is the freely available Saarbruecken Voice Database (SVD) in which voices were sampled at 50 kHz with 16-bit resolution in the same environment. Here only vowels in SVD are used in the multi-view learning. Thereafter, each audio is denoted by the name of the vowel and the adopted pitch. "a-n," for example, is the vowel /a/ pronounced at a normal pitch. Here, we use a set $V = \{$a-n, a-l, a-h, a-lhl, i-n, i-l, i-h, i-lhl, u-n, u-l, u-h, u-lhl$\}$ to denote all vowels.

In this section, we conduct two classification tasks: (1) healthy versus recurrent laryngeal nerve paralysis (RLNP) and (2) healthy versus spasmodic dysphonia (SD). Clearly, the problem of class imbalance occurs in the detection of both RLNP and SD. In this case, accuracy rate (*Acc*) and three other metrics are used for evaluation, which are sensitivity (*Sen*), specificity (*Spe*), and the geometric mean (*Gmean*) of *Sen* and *Spe*. The four metrics are defined with Eqs. (7.22)–(7.25), with the TP, TN, FP, and FN explained in Table 7.1. More discussions on the metrics for imbalanced data can be found in Lopez et al. (2013).

$$\text{Sen} = \frac{\text{TP}}{\text{TP} + \text{FN}} \tag{7.22}$$

$$\text{Spe} = \frac{\text{TN}}{\text{FP} + \text{TN}}. \tag{7.23}$$

$$\text{Acc} = \frac{\text{TN} + \text{TP}}{\text{FP} + \text{TN} + \text{TP} + \text{FN}}. \tag{7.24}$$

$$\text{Gmean} = \sqrt{\text{Sen} \times \text{Spe}}. \tag{7.25}$$

In the two classification tasks, we compare the performance of our approach with that of three baselines.

1. $1NN_{sBest}$: the result using classifier 1-NN on the most informative audio, i.e., one that achieves the best performance (highest *Gmean*).

Table 7.1 Confusion matrix for a two-class problem

	Disease prediction	Health prediction
Disease class	True positive (TP)	False negative (FN)
Health class	False positive (FP)	True negative (TN)

2. INN_{comb}: this method concatenates features of all audios and then applies the classifier 1-NN.
3. *MCCA*: the multi-view canonical correlation analysis (MCCA) (Kettenring 1971), which analyzes linear relations among multi-view, is one of the classical feature fusion methods. For fair comparison with our method ROME-DLR, the same classifier 1-NN follows.

For all methods in the comparison, fivefold cross-validation is conducted and repeated 50 times, whose results are represented by "mean ± standard deviation %." Note that the ADASYN strategy handling class imbalance of training set is performed for all methods in the comparison.

7.3.2 The Detection of RLNP

Flaccidity of vocal fold and dysphonia, common symptoms for patients with RLNP (Crumley 1994), causes perturbation of fundamental frequency and amplitude of voice over periods. Hence, jitter and shimmer having 22 variants are used as features in the detection of RLNP (Tsanas 2012). Then principal component analysis (PCA) follows to reduce the high correlation, where the reduced dimensionality is estimated by the maximum likelihood method (Levina and Bickel 2005).

The model parameters α, β, τ, and λ are specified empirically as 0.005, 0.01, 0.1, and 0.5, respectively. Table 7.2 shows the performance of RLNP detection when all 12 vowels are used in the fusion. Overall, our method ROME-DLR obtains the highest *Acc*, *Gmean*, and *Sen*, whereas it achieves the second highest *Spe* by a margin of 0.8% points.

In detail, the $1NN_{sBest}$ gives the worst performance, showing that multi-view fusion is generally beneficial. The $1NN_{comb}$ achieves the lowest sensitivity rate but the highest specificity rate. Clearly, the method $1NN_{comb}$ tends to classify most samples to the healthy class. Even though MCCA considers the linear relations between different views, its projected features are not discriminative since its projection matrices are learned in an unsupervised manner.

In contrast, ROME-DLR considers the shared-specific structures in the multi-view data and adopts the regression model to make full use of the label information. As shown, ROME-DLR indeed outperforms MCCA regarding all four metrics. Therefore, the superiority of ROME-DLR in RLNP detection is demonstrated.

In addition, we also evaluate the proposed method when the number of audios participating in fusion varies from 2 to 11. Altogether, the result is illustrated in

Table 7.2 Performance of different models in RLNP detection when all 12 vowels are used for fusion

Models	Acc (%)	Gmean (%)	Sen (%)	Spe (%)
$1NN_{sBest}$	73.02 ± 1.13	64.99 ± 1.37	54.25 ± 2.05	78.36 ± 1.32
$1NN_{comb}$	76.39 ± 3.04	63.84 ± 4.96	48.71 ± 7.52	**84.27 ± 3.62**
MCCA	76.46 ± 3.01	70.30 ± 4.72	61.64 ± 8.47	80.67 ± 3.76
ROME-DLR	**81.58 ± 2.78**	**78.97 ± 3.81**	**74.94 ± 7.02**	83.47 ± 3.35

Bold values indicate better results

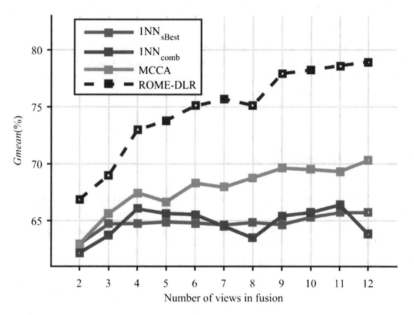

Fig. 7.1 (color online) *Gmean* versus different numbers of audios participating in fusion in RLNP detection

Fig. 7.1. For briefness, the performance is measured with *Gmean* only, which is a trade-off between *Sen* and *Spe* and thus being a reasonable metric for class imbalanced data. Without loss of generality, when the view number is *i* in Fig. 7.1, it means that the first *i* audios in set *V* are used in fusion. Clearly, ROME-DLR achieves the highest *Gmean* for all view numbers. In particular, the advantage is more significant when the view number is over 8. With the increase of view number, the *Gmean* rate of ROME-DLR is almost monotonically increasing, which is beneficial since it implies that there is no need to optimize the view number.

7.3.3   The Detection of SD

SD disease starts at the base of brain, which regulates involuntary muscle movement (Kirke et al. 2017). For patients with SD, their pronounced voice is abnormal. Due to inaccurate muscle movements in vocal tract, MFCC related features are used. We first compute the MFCC coefficients, delta-coefficients and delta-delta coefficients for each frame in an audio. Finally, each audio is represented with the standard deviations (*std*) of MFCC over all frames, *std* of delta-coefficients, and *std* of delta-delta coefficients. Finally, as in Sect. 7.3.2, PCA follows to reduce correlation between features.

Empirically, parameters α, β, τ, and λ in our model are specified as 0.1, 0.05, 0.005, and 0.6, respectively. The results of detecting SD with all 12 vowels are given in Table 7.3. As shown, using the proposed ROME-DLR model to fuse different audios is still beneficial as it achieves the highest *Acc*, *Gmean*, and *Spe*. Again, ROME-DLR is superior to the MCCA method in terms of all four metrics. Besides, the sensitivity and specificity rates of ROME-DLR are both over 91%, making ROME-DLR a possible model to detect SD detection in clinical setting.

Additionally, the comparison is also conducted when the view number ranges from 2 to 11, as presented in Fig. 7.2. Again, the ROME-DLR achieves a higher *Gmean* rate than that of other models and leads to good performance even with fewer audios. Besides, the projected features by ROME-DLR are more discriminative due to the exploiting of label information.

7.3.4   Ablation Study

Due to limited space, we only give the analysis of ROME-DLR when it is used for the fusion of 12 vowels in SD detection. The adopted measure is *Gmean*.

7.3.4.1   Regularization Parameters α and β

First, we investigate the sensitivity of parameters α and β in ROME-DLR. The values of both parameters α and β are changed within the range of $\{0, 0.001, 0.005, 0.01, 0.05, 0.1, 0.5, 1\}$. Figure 7.3 illustrates the *Gmean* versus the different values

Table 7.3 Performance of different models in SD detection when all 12 vowels are used for fusion

Models	Acc (%)	Gmean (%)	Sen (%)	Spe (%)
$1NN_{sBest}$	87.86 ± 0.76	70.48 ± 2.58	55.47 ± 3.82	90.79 ± 0.68
$1NN_{comb}$	74.70 ± 5.08	82.38 ± 4.12	93.24 ± 6.71	73.02 ± 5.59
MCCA	90.89 ± 2.27	89.33 ± 4.86	87.82 ± 9.26	91.16 ± 2.41
ROME-DLR	$\mathbf{92.29 \pm 1.93}$	$\mathbf{91.69 \pm 4.22}$	$\mathbf{91.20 \pm 8.07}$	$\mathbf{92.39 \pm 2.02}$

Bold values indicate better results

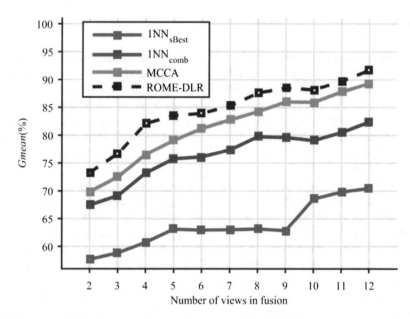

Fig. 7.2 (color online) *Gmean* versus different numbers of audios participating in fusion in SD detection

of α and β. The deeper the color is, the higher the *Gmean* is. Generally, we find that large β leads to an inferior performance, as seen in the bottom two rows. Similarly, shared components are less discovered with a larger α. A proper balance between α and β is necessary to find the actual shared-specific structures hidden in each dataset. However, when β takes the values of 0.01 and 0.05, and α is smaller (6 0.5), the performance remains relatively stable, which shows that ROME-DLR is insensitive to the parameters α and β in a reasonable range. From Fig. 7.3, the optimal α and β are set as 0.1 and 0.05, respectively.

7.3.4.2   Parameter τ

Parameter τ is a penalty constant that controls the difference between shared component and the average of the view-specific components. In this part, we evaluate its influence by setting τ as 0, 0.001, 0.005, 0.01, 0.05, 0.1, 0.5, and 1, respectively, and then report the achieved *Gmean* in Table 7.4. As shown, the model performs the best when $\tau = 0.005$. In particular, the *Gmean* rate decreases when τ is larger than 0.05. On the other hand, when τ is zero and thus the penalty term is not used, lower *Gmean* rate is achieved. Hence, a proper τ is necessary.

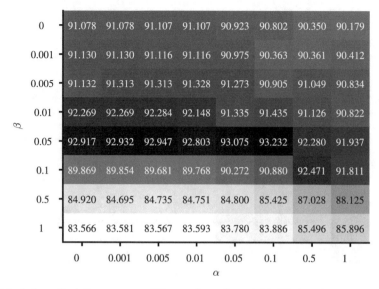

Fig. 7.3 (color online) *Gmean* versus different values of α and β in SD detection

Table 7.4 Effects of parameter τ on classification (%)

Parameter τ	0	0.001	0.005	0.01	0.05	0.1	0.5	1
Gmean (%)	92.81	92.81	**92.84**	92.71	92.58	92.46	92.07	91.80

Bold values indicate better results

7.3.4.3 Parameter λ

In ROME-DLR, the parameter λ is introduced to control the balance between the shared matrix W_0 and the view-specific component W_i ($i = 1, 2, \cdots, m$). Here, we investigate its influence by varying it from 0 to 1 with a step size of 0.1. The results are presented in Fig. 7.4. Generally, with the increase of λ, the *Gmean* rate firstly increases and then decreases. Therefore, the optimal value of λ is assigned as 0.6. Specially, when λ equals to 1, the *Gmean* rate is 8.2% points lower than the highest rate. Meanwhile, the performance decreases 1.39% points when λ is 0 (no shared structure is modeled). Therefore, the balance between shared and specific structures is important to achieve better performance. Note that a good trade-off between α and β, a proper τ, and an appropriate λ are all necessary to explore the actual hidden shared-specific structures in multi-view data.

7.3.4.4 The Influence of ADASYN

ADASYN is utilized to handle the class imbalance problem in SD detection. The results with and without ADASYN are presented in Table 7.5. When no ADASYN

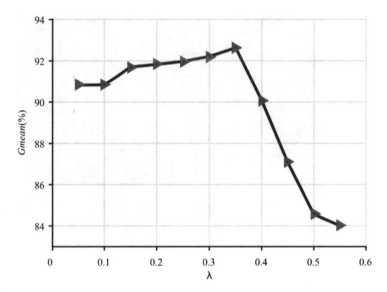

Fig. 7.4 (color online) *Gmean* versus different values of λ in SD detection

Table 7.5 The results with and without ADASYN

ADASYN	Acc (%)	Gmean (%)	Sen (%)	Spe (%)
No	**93.81 ± 1.74**	81.51 ± 7.76	69.87 ± 12.91	**95.98 ± 1.62**
Yes	92.23 ± 2.2	**91.72 ± 4.54**	**91.37 ± 8.56**	92.32 ± 2.32

Bold values indicate better results

is used, the *Sen* rate is quite low, indicating that most samples of interest (patients with SD) are classified as healthy. In contrast, after using ADASYN on training set, the *Sen* rate increases over 21% points while the *Spe* rate drops around 4% points. The increase of the *Gmean* rate demonstrates the overall improvement. Therefore, special attention is needed when ROME-DLR is used in class imbalanced classification tasks, especially in many clinical settings.

7.4   Discussions

In ROME-DLR, the feature vector of view i for each sample is transformed into a c-dimensional vector using projection matrices W_i and W_0. We visualize the transformed features in an instance to demonstrate the effectiveness of the proposed method. In Fig. 7.5, the left one shows the first two principal components (from a PCA analysis) of the original features of the first audio ("a-n"), while the right plot illustrates the two-dimensional features generated with $X_1^T(\lambda W_0 + (1 - \lambda)W_1)$, where the transformed matrices W_1 and W_0 are learned jointly by ROME-DLR

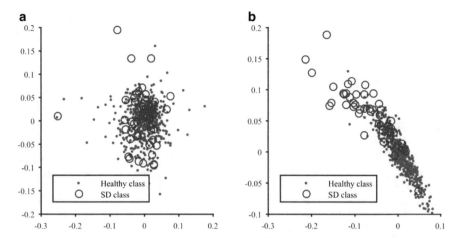

Fig. 7.5 (color online) The visualization of the original features (first two principal components) and the features generated by ROME-DLR. (**a**) the original features. (**b**) the generated features

using all 12 views in *V*. The transformed features of the same class show more compact distribution. Moreover, comparing with Fig. 7.5a, the red dot and blue circle are more separable in Fig. 7.5b, indicating that the transformed features are more discriminative. Overall, the small within-class variation and large between-class distance substantiate the superiority of the proposed learning approach.

We must point out that many kinds of classifier, such as the nearest neighbor (1-NN), support vector machine (SVM) and random forest (RF), can be used for the final classification in ROME-DLR. Additionally, since ROME-DLR uses feature matrices as input, this model is also applicable to the fusion of other modalities other than audio.

7.5   Summary

In this chapter, we propose a regression based model ROME-DLR to fuse features from different audios for disease detection. Unlike existing methods which use a single audio or simply concatenate audios or features together for fusion, the proposed method considers the correlation among different audios and exploits the label information to learn discriminative projections. Particularly, we assume a shared-specific structure in multi-view data to uncover the correlation among different audios. Then the traditional binary regression targets are relaxed to be more flexible and margins between different classes can be enlarged, which enables more discriminative projections. We further adopt the $l_{2,1}$ norm on the regression term to handle possible noise and outliers. The presented method is optimized with an efficient algorithm and experiments on two detection tasks (with varying number of audios for fusion) substantiate the effectiveness and superiority of our method.

Our algorithm may provide motivation to explore fusion of multi-audio for the detection of other diseases. However, the ROME-DLR model can only deal with homogenous features. In the future, we may investigate the fusion when features of different audios are heterogeneous.

References

Arias-Londono, J. D., Godino-Llorente, J. I., Saenz-Lechn, N., Osma-Ruiz, V., & Castellanos-Dominguez, G. (2010). An improved method for voice pathology detection by means of a HMM-based feature space transformation. *Pattern Recogn.*, *43*, 3100 – 3112.

Brabanter, K. D., Karsmakers, P., Brabanter, J. D., Suykens, J., & Moor, B. D. (2012). Confidence bands for least squares support vector machine classifiers: A regression approach. *Pattern Recogn.*, *45*, 2280 – 2287. Brain Decoding.

Childers, D. G., & Bae, K. S. (1992). Detection of laryngeal function using speech and electroglottographic data. *IEEE Trans. Biomed. Eng.*, *39*, 19–25.

Crumley, R. L. (1994). Unilateral recurrent laryngeal nerve paralysis. *J. Voice*, *8*, 79–83.

Garcia, J. O., & Garcia, C. R. (2003). Mel-frequency cepstrum coefficients extraction from infant cry for classification of normal and pathological cry with feed-forward neural networks. In *Neural Networks, 2003. Proceedings of the International Joint Conference on* (pp. 3140–3145). IEEE volume 4.

Gestel, T. V., Suykens, J. A., Lanckriet, G., Lambrechts, A., Moor, B. D., & Vandewalle, J. (2002). Bayesian framework for least-squares support vector machine classifiers, Gaussian processes, and kernel fisher discriminant analysis. *Neural Comput.*, *14*, 1115–1147.

Ghasemishabankareh, B., Li, X., & Ozlen, M. (2016). Cooperative coevolutionary differential evolution with improved augmented Lagrangian to solve constrained optimisation problems. *Inf. Sci.*, *369*, 441–456.

Godino-Llorente, J. I., & Gomez-Vilda, P. (2004). Automatic detection of voice impairments by means of short-term cepstral parameters and neural network based detectors. *IEEE Trans. Biomed. Eng.*, *51*, 380–384.

Godino-Llorente, J. I., Gomez-Vilda, P., & Blanco-Velasco, M. (2006). Dimensionality reduction of a pathological voice quality assessment system based on Gaussian mixture models and short-term cepstral parameters. *IEEE Trans. Biomed. Eng.*, *53*, 1943–1953.

He, H., Bai, Y., Garcia, E. A., & Li, S. (2008). ADASYN: Adaptive synthetic sampling approach for imbalanced learning. In *Neural Networks, 2008. IJCNN 2008. (IEEE World Congress on Computational Intelligence). IEEE International Joint Conference on* (pp. 1322–1328). IEEE.

Hu, J.-F., Zheng, W.-S., Lai, J., & Zhang, J. (2015). Jointly learning heterogeneous features for RGB-D activity recognition. In *Computer Vision and Pattern Recognition (CVPR), 2015 IEEE Conference on* (pp. 5344–5352). IEEE.

Lopez-de Ipina, K., Alonso, J.-B., Travieso, C. M., Sole-Casals, J., Egiraun, H., Faundez-Zanuy, M., Ezeiza, A., Barroso, N., Ecay-Torres, M., MartinezLage, P. et al. (2013). On the selection of non-invasive methods based on speech analysis oriented to automatic Alzheimer disease diagnosis. *Sensors*, *13*, 6730–6745.

Izenman, A. J. (2008). Modern multivariate statistical techniques. *Regression, classification and manifold learning.*

Jotz, G. P., Cervantes, O., Abrahao, M., Settanni, F. A. P., & de Angelis, E. C. (2002). Noise-to-harmonics ratio as an acoustic measure of voice disorders in boys. *J. Voice*, *16*, 28–31.

Kettenring, J. R. (1971). Canonical analysis of several sets of variables. *Biometrika*, *58*, 433–451.

Kirke, D. N., Battistella, G., Kumar, V., Rubien-Thomas, E., Choy, M., Rumbach, A., & Simonyan, K. (2017). Neural correlates of dystonic tremor: a multimodal study of voice tremor in spasmodic dysphonia. *Brain Imaging Behav.*, *11*, 166–175.

Kong, D., Ding, C., & Huang, H. (2011). Robust nonnegative matrix factorization using l21-norm. In *Proceedings of the 20th ACM international conference on Information and knowledge management* (pp. 673–682). ACM.

Levina, E., & Bickel, P. J. (2005). Maximum likelihood estimation of intrinsic dimension. In *Advances in neural information processing systems* (pp. 777– 784).

Li, J., Zhang, D., Li, Y., Wu, J., & Zhang, B. (2017). Joint similar and specific learning for diabetes mellitus and impaired glucose regulation detection. *Inf. Sci.*, *384*, 191–204.

Little, M. A., McSharry, P. E., Hunter, E. J., Spielman, J., Ramig, L. O. et al. (2009). Suitability of dysphonia measurements for telemonitoring of Parkinson's disease. *IEEE Trans. Biomed. Eng.*, *56*, 1015–1022.

Little, M. A., McSharry, P. E., Roberts, S. J., Costello, D. A., & Moroz, I. M. (2007). Exploiting nonlinear recurrence and fractal scaling properties for voice disorder detection. *Biomed. Eng. Online*, *6*, 23.

Lopez, V., Fernandez, A., Garcia, S., Palade, V., & Herrera, F. (2013). An insight into classification with imbalanced data: Empirical results and current trends on using data intrinsic characteristics. *Inf. Sci.*, *250*, 113–141.

Ludlow, C., Bassich, C., Connor, N., Coulter, D., Lee, Y., Baer, T., Sasaki, C., & Harris, K. (1987). The validity of using phonatory jitter and shimmer to detect laryngeal pathology. In *Laryngeal function in phonation and respiration* (pp. 492–508). College-Hill Press, Boston.

Maciel, C. D., Guido, R. C., Fonseca, E. S., Montagnoli, A. N., & Vieira, L. S. (2007). Autoregressive decomposition and pole tracking applied to vocal fold nodule signals. *Pattern Recogn. Lett.*, *28*, 1360–1367.

Martinez, D., Lleida, E., Ortega, A., & Miguel, A. (2012a). Score level versus audio level fusion for voice pathology detection on the Saarbrucken Voice Database. In *Advances in Speech and Language Technologies for Iberian Languages* (pp. 110–120). Berlin, Heidelberg: Springer Berlin Heidelberg.

Martinez, D., Lleida, E., Ortega, A., Miguel, A., & Villalba, J. (2012b). Voice pathology detection on the Saarbrucken Voice Database with calibration and fusion of scores using multifocal toolkit. In *Advances in Speech and Language Technologies for Iberian Languages* (pp. 99–109). Berlin, Heidelberg: Springer Berlin Heidelberg.

Maryn, Y., Corthals, P., Van Cauwenberge, P., Roy, N., & De Bodt, M. (2010). Toward improved ecological validity in the acoustic measurement of overall voice quality: combining continuous speech and sustained vowels. *J. Voice*, *24*, 540–555.

Nie, F., Huang, H., Cai, X., & Ding, C. H. (2010). Efficient and robust feature selection via joint 2, 1-norms minimization. In *Advances in neural information processing systems* (pp. 1813–1821).

Oguz, H., Demirci, M., Safak, M. A., Arslan, N., Islam, A., & Kargin, S. (2007). Effects of unilateral vocal cord paralysis on objective voice measures obtained by Praat. *Eur. Arch. Oto-Rhino-Laryn.*, *264*, 257–261.

Orozco-Arroyave, J., Honig, F., Arias-Londono, J., Vargas-Bonilla, J., Daqrouq, K., Skodda, S., Rusz, J., & Noth, E. (2016). Automatic detection of Parkinson's disease in running speech spoken in three different languages. *J. Acoust. Soc. Am.*, *139*, 481–500.

Ren, C.-X., Dai, D.-Q., & Yan, H. (2012). Robust classification using 2, 1- norm based regression model. *Pattern Recogn.*, *45*, 2708–2718.

Saldanha, J. C., Ananthakrishna, T., & Pinto, R. (2014). Vocal fold pathology assessment using Mel-frequency cepstral coefficients and linear predictive cepstral coefficients features. *J. Med. Imaging Health Inform.*, *4*, 168–173.

Saudi, A. S. M., Youssif, A. A., & Ghalwash, A. Z. (2012). Computer aided recognition of vocal folds disorders by means of RASTA-PLP. *Comput. Inf. Sci.*, *5*, 39.

Shi, Y., Suk, H.-I., Gao, Y., & Shen, D. (2014). Joint coupled-feature representation and coupled boosting for ad diagnosis. In *Proceedings of the IEEE Conference on Computer Vision and Pattern Recognition* (pp. 2721–2728).

Shin, D., Lee, H. S., & Kim, D. (2007). Illumination-robust face recognition using ridge regressive bilinear models. *Pattern Recogn. Lett.*, *29*, 49–58.

Tsanas, A. (2012). *Accurate telemonitoring of Parkinson's disease symptom severity using nonlinear speech signal processing and statistical machine learning*. Ph.D. thesis University of Oxford.

Tsanas, A., Little, M. A., McSharry, P. E., & Ramig, L. O. (2010). Accurate telemonitoring of Parkinson's disease progression by noninvasive speech tests. *IEEE Trans. Biomed. Eng.*, *57*, 884–893.

Tsanas, A., Little, M. A., McSharry, P. E., Spielman, J., & Ramig, L. O. (2012). Novel speech signal processing algorithms for high-accuracy classification of Parkinson's disease. *IEEE Trans. Biomed. Eng.*, *59*, 1264–1271.

Vaiciukynas, E., Verikas, A., Gelzinis, A., Bacauskiene, M., Kons, Z., Satt, A., & Hoory, R. (2014). Fusion of voice signal information for detection of mild laryngeal pathology. *Appl. Soft. Comput.*, *18*, 91–103.

Vaiciukynas, E., Verikas, A., Gelzinis, A., Bacauskiene, M., Vaskevicius, K., Uloza, V., Padervinskis, E., & Ciceliene, J. (2016). Fusing various audio feature sets for detection of Parkinson's disease from sustained voice and speech recordings. In *International Conference on Speech and Computer* (pp. 328 – 337). Springer.

Xiang, S., Nie, F., Meng, G., Pan, C., & Zhang, C. (2012). Discriminative least squares regression for multiclass classification and feature selection. *IEEE Trans. Neural Netw. Learn.*, *23*, 1738–1754.

Xue, H., Chen, S., & Yang, Q. (2009). Discriminatively regularized least-squares classification. *Pattern Recogn.*, *42*, 93–104.

Yang, M., Zhang, L., Zhang, D., & Wang, S. (2012). Relaxed collaborative representation for pattern classification. In *Computer Vision and Pattern Recognition (CVPR), 2012 IEEE Conference on* (pp. 2224–2231). IEEE.

Yumoto, E., Gould, W. J., & Baer, T. (1982). Harmonics-to-noise ratio as an index of the degree of hoarseness. *J. Acoust. Soc. Am.*, *71*, 1544–1550.

Zhang, X.-Y., Wang, L., Xiang, S., & Liu, C.-L. (2015). Retargeted least squares regression algorithm. *IEEE Trans. Neural Netw. Learn.*, *26*, 2206–2213.

Chapter 8
Book Review and Future Work

Abstract With the title "Pathological voice analysis," this book mainly focuses on the building models for the analysis of pathological voice. The book contains three parts. Firstly, a brief overview of pathological voice analysis and a guideline on the voice acquisition for clinical use are presented. Secondly, we introduce two important signal processing steps in pathological voice analysis, which are pitch estimation and glottal closure instants (GCI) detection. Finally, feature learning and the multi-audio fusion are shown for discriminating pathological voice from the healthy ones. In this chapter, we summarize the book and present future work for pathological voice analysis. Section 8.1 gives an overview of the previous chapters. In Sect. 8.2, we discuss the future work in pathological voice analysis.

Keywords Book review · Future work

8.1 Book Recapitulation

With the rapid development of artificial intelligence, there have been more and more works that try to apply this technology to medical field. Although voice is a typical biomedical signal, most studies based on voice still focus on speaker and speech recognition. In this book, we present our recent researches on pathological voice analysis which is based on the theory of signal processing and machine learning.

Chapter 1 first introduces the research background and significance of pathological voice analysis, in which the biomedical value of voice is particularly emphasized and the systematic review of pathological voice analysis is presented. In addition, challenges in the pathological voice analysis are discussed from three aspects: data layer, feature layer, and model layer.

In Chap. 2, the influence of sampling rate for pathological voice analysis is studied. First of all, we build a dataset of different sampling rate. Then six different metrics, which are information entropy, reconstruction error, feature correlation, classification accuracy, computational cost, and storage cost, are adopted to experiment the influence of sampling rate on voice based disease detection. With these

© Springer Nature Singapore Pte Ltd. 2020
D. Zhang, K. Wu, *Pathological Voice Analysis*,
https://doi.org/10.1007/978-981-32-9196-6_8

extensive devised experiments, we show a guideline on how to choose sampling rate for pathological voice analysis.

The next two chapters present two signal processing methods that are essential for pathological voice analysis. In Chap. 3, a harmonic enhancement based pitch estimation algorithm is studied since many key features in pathological voice analysis depend on the exact pitch estimation. First, we analyze the existing pitch extraction algorithm and point out that missing and submerged harmonics are the root causes for the failures of many pitch detectors, especially for pathological voice. Then a novel direction is put forward, which is to improve harmonics structures before implementing the pitch detection. Meanwhile, a detailed harmonic enhancement method is introduced based on the Fourier transform theory. Experimental results show that the proposed algorithm can effectively reduce the error rate of pitch detection and it can be used for other periodic signals.

Chapter 4 presents a glottal closure instant (GCI) detection method that is applicable for pathological voice. Due to the local discontinuities and nonlinearity in pathological voice, we propose to use the nonlinear instantaneous speech energy operator TKEO (Teager–Kaiser energy operator) for GCI extraction and adopt multiresolution fusion strategies to enhance the performance. Experimental results show that the algorithm has low computational complexity, does not rely on pitch information, and its performance is particularly advantageous for noisy and pathological voice. Besides, the relation between TKEO and second derivative operator is revealed, which is that operator TKEO can be approximately regarded as the local-mean-weighted second derivative.

In Chap. 5, feature extraction in pathological voice analysis is discussed. Different from traditional hand-crafted features, a feature learning algorithm based on the first derivative of the Mel spectrum is presented. This data-driven algorithm adopts clustering methods to train encoding dictionaries for healthy voice and pathological voice, respectively, and then encodes the voice signal with the resulting dictionaries to obtain the learned features. Compared with the traditional handed-design features, the presented algorithm can greatly improve the performance of pathological voice detection and provides useful conclusions for feature learning and design.

In order to make full use of all the audio collected for each subject, Chaps. 6 and 7 analyze the problem of multi-audio fusion from the perspective of model layer. In Chap. 6, we develop a two-audio joint learning algorithm JOLL4R that is based on residual coupling. This algorithm enables the two audios to cooperate with each other so that a larger weight can be adaptively assigned to the audio that is more discriminative. In Chap. 7, we also propose a robust discriminative analysis algorithm ROME-DLR by mining the shared-specific structure in multi-audio data. This method decomposes each audio into shared component and specific component, in which the shared one is to express the similarity between multiple audios to enhance the stability of our algorithm, while the latter one retains the uniqueness of each audio for complementary purpose. At the same time, the algorithm also uses the $l_{2,1}$ norm to measure the regression residual in order to gain robustness against outliers. Experimental results show that the above two audio fusion algorithms can improve the performance of pathological voice detection significantly.

8.2 Future Work

With the proposed algorithms in previous chapters, some aspects in pathological voice analysis are studied and discussed, such as data sampling, pitch estimation, glottal closure instant detection, feature learning, and multi-audio fusion for pathological voice. In the future, the directions worth further exploring are listed in the following:

1. Extend the proposed algorithms to other applications
   The fundamental frequency extraction algorithm iPEEH and the period segmentation algorithm GMAT presented in the book have been successfully used in the analysis of pathological voice. In fact, these algorithms are applicable in speech synthesis applications, which may be needed by patients with pathological voice. In addition, these algorithms can be used in other periodic or quasi-periodic signals such as EEG and ECG in the future. Since the input of the fusion algorithms JOLL4R and ROME-DLR proposed in Chaps. 6 and 7 are extracted features, thus these algorithms can also be used in other modal fusion applications.
2. Pathological voice analysis based on deep learning
   Deep learning method can mine features of different abstraction levels, and it has achieved success in many fields such as face recognition and speech recognition. In the further exploration of pathological voice analysis, deep learning may play an important role. In particular, the small sample size problem, which is a significant challenge in pathological voice analysis as pointed out in Chap. 1, may be alleviated by adopting transfer learning strategy in deep learning. The so-called transfer learning is to transfer the trained model parameters to the relevant new model to improve the performance of the new model by reducing overfitting. For example, Bar et al. proposed to use a convolutional neural network (CNN) trained on ImageNet (Deng et al. 2009), which is a non-medical image dataset, for disease detection based on chest X-ray and achieved good results (Bar et al. 2015). Similarly, Ng et al. used the CNN network trained on ImageNet to recognize facial expressions (Ng et al. 2015). In particular, we may try to transfer a deep learning model trained for speech recognition (speaker recognition) model to pathological voice analysis.
3. Joint analysis with other biomedical signals
   In order to improve the performance of disease detection and tracking, a variety of biomedical signals including voice can be analyzed jointly. For example, patients with Parkinson's disease often suffer from motor disorders, researchers have attempted to use their handwriting (Zhi et al. 2015) and gait (using wearable accelerometers) (Mazilu et al. 2012) for quantitative measurements of their condition. Therefore, we may analyze the voice and motor related signals jointly so as to detect and monitor the disease more comprehensively and accurately.

References

Bar, Y., Diamant, I., Wolf, L., Lieberman, S., Konen, E., & Greenspan, H. (2015). Chest pathology detection using deep learning with non-medical training. In *IEEE International Symposium on Biomedical Imaging. IEEE*.

Deng, J., Dong, W., Socher, R., Li, L. J., & Li, F. F. (2009). ImageNet: a Large-Scale Hierarchical Image Database. In *IEEE Computer Society Conference on Computer Vision and Pattern Recognition, 20-25 June 2009, USA. IEEE*.

Mazilu, S., Hardegger, M., Zhu, Z., Roggen, D., & Hausdorff, J. M. (2012). Online Detection of Freezing of Gait with Smartphones and Machine Learning Techniques. In *Pervasive Computing Technologies for Healthcare, 2012 6th International Conference on. IEEE*.

Ng, H. W., Nguyen, D., Vonikakis, V., & Winkler, S. (2015). Deep Learning for Emotion Recognition on Small Datasets Using Transfer Learning. In *ACM International Conference on Multimodal Interaction. ACM*.

Zhi, N., Jaeger, B. K., Gouldstone, A., Frank, S., & Sipahi, R. (2015). Objective Quantitative Assessment of Movement Disorders Through Analysis of Static Handwritten Characters. In *ASME Dynamic Systems & Control Conference*.

Index

© Springer Nature Singapore Pte Ltd. 2020
D. Zhang, K. Wu, *Pathological Voice Analysis*,
https://doi.org/10.1007/978-981-32-9196-6